Orgasms
and how to
have them

Orgasms

and how to have them

a guide for women

Jenny Hare

First published in Great Britain in 2007 by Fusion Press,
a division of Satin Publications Ltd
101 Southwark Street
London SE1 0JF
UK
info@visionpaperbacks.co.uk
www.visionpaperbacks.co.uk
Publisher: Sheena Dewan

A catalogue record for this book is available from the British Library.

ISBN-13: 978-1-905745-04-3

2 4 6 8 10 9 7 5 3 1

Cover and text design by ok?design
Printed and bound in the UK by
Mackays of Chatham Ltd, Chatham, Kent

Contents

Acknowledgements   ix

Introduction   I

Chapter 1: What is an Orgasm?   4

Chapter 2: Loving Yourself, Loving Your Body   24

Chapter 3: How to Have an Orgasm on Your Own   42

Chapter 4: Once You Get Going – Variations on a Theme   66

Chapter 5: How to Have an Orgasm with a Partner   84

Chapter 6: Making a Relationship a Great Place for Orgasms   134

Chapter 7: Health and Well-Being   173

Chapter 8: Why am I Still Not Orgasming?   223

A Final Note   239

Useful Resources   242

About the Author   246

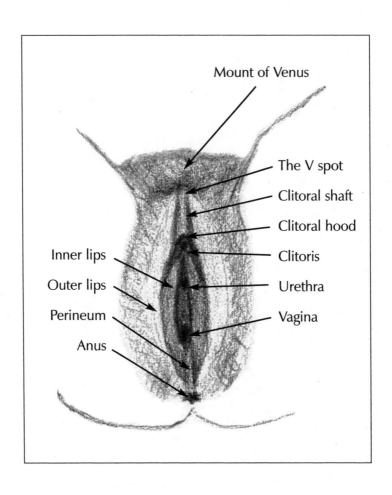

Mount of Venus

The V spot

Clitoral shaft

Clitoral hood

Inner lips

Clitoris

Outer lips

Urethra

Perineum

Vagina

Anus

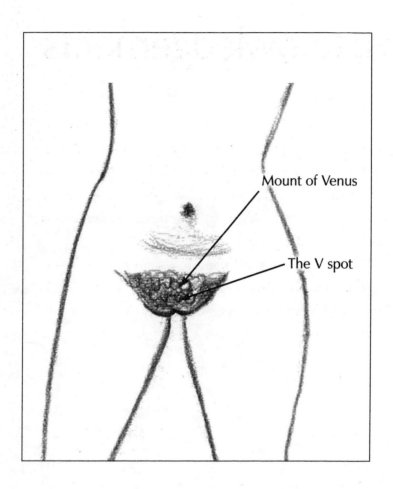

Acknowledgements

My thanks to everyone who has been involved with this book at Vision, especially Kate Pollard, for her insights, thoroughness and encouragement. Also thanks to my agent, Charlotte Howard, for urging me to write this book in the first place.

And, as ever, my thanks and love to my sister, Penny Stanway, and to all my friends for bearing with me while I was engrossed in the book for so many months!

Introduction

Since gaining sexual freedom in the 1960s, the double standards regarding sex have almost disappeared for women. And with effective contraceptives allowing us to have sex without the fear of pregnancy, we're all having a wonderfully fulfilling time.

Sounds fantastic, doesn't it? But are we *really* having great sex? Sadly the answer for many women is still no. The fact is, most women don't have brilliant sex lives and, in reality, many of us get precious little satisfaction because we experience problems climaxing. Exactly how many women are affected? Surveys indicate that a high percentage of us (at least one in ten) have *never* had an orgasm, while many more have currently lost the knack completely (around 30 per cent) and another 40 per cent can't rely on having an orgasm most times they have sex. So, at best, only one in five women is confident of having an orgasm easily when she wants one. Take into account the many women who are shy of admitting they can't have orgasms and we're talking about the vast majority of us missing out on one of life's joys.

Over many years as a sex therapist, counsellor and agony aunt, I've encouraged women to discover their orgasmability. What I've learnt from listening to their personal stories is that the reasons for their difficulty in climaxing are many and varied, and that often several combine to snarl up their innate ability.

I wanted to write this book to offer clear guidelines to every woman who wishes to learn, rediscover or practise how to be easily orgasmic and how to confidently have an orgasm whenever she wants. So if you're not having orgasms just now, find it difficult or unreliable or have never had one, this book will show you how to discover the knack.

For simplicity regarding relationships I've mostly referred to heterosexual ones throughout the book, but other than the sections on intercourse, the book is just as apt for lesbians.

Because we're such complex creatures, our minds, emotions or a clog in the physical works can all too easily inhibit our ability to enjoy sex or have orgasms. Each woman's story is individual, so your discovery process of what's stopping you from having orgasms will be too. Very likely it's something as straightforward as learning

Introduction

a good orgasmic technique, but other things could be impacting on your orgasmability.

The book has been arranged in a step-by-step order, first explaining how an orgasm works, then how to have one in or out of a relationship and finally how to troubleshoot anything stopping you from climaxing. If you prefer to read the book intuitively and flick straight to the chapters or sections where you sense you'll find the information you personally need, that's fine. Your story is individual and your discovery process will be too. But as the learning curve about orgasm is fascinating and our scope for having different kinds and levels of orgasm are very wide, I hope that even if you become orgasmic soon – or better still straight away – you'll be drawn to read more of the book.

Keep the thought of an easy pleasure path to orgasm in mind and never feel daunted as once any causes or 'blocks' are resolved or removed, you can confidently expect to become orgasmic and, once it starts to happen for you, it will soon become natural and easy.

Being orgasmic is not always, of course, necessary for great sex – some women have a wonderful, deeply satisfying time making love to themselves or a partner even though it doesn't end in climax. This book is for the vast majority who aren't easily orgasmic and want to be. I hope it will expand your pleasure and enable you to be orgasmic.

Chapter 1

What is an Orgasm?

Orgasms are as varied as our personalities. No one knows, of course, how other women's experiences compare to our own, but just as we presume that we see the same colours as most others do, so we can assume that we have largely similar experiences of orgasm as other women. Having said that, we can have distinctly differing kinds of orgasm depending on variables such as the amount or kind of arousal, our phase of life, hormone cycles, mood and health.

A crescendo of highly pleasurable sensations in and around the clitoris and/or vagina is the essence of the first stage of orgasm. Then there is a feeling of going over the brink at the top of that crescendo and letting go to an extreme pleasure unlike any other – this is the central, most intense part. On a more complex level it can encompass a surge of euphoric feelings.

Are there different types of orgasm?

Much has been said and written about the location of an orgasm. Many years ago it was tacitly accepted that it happened in the vagina, but in the 1960s the clitoris came into focus and women, on trying to work out precisely where the sensation occurred, came to the general conclusion that the clitoris, as well as being the orchestrator of climax, was also where we experienced it. Later, the concept of the G spot and vaginal orgasm came back into fashion. In this book I also talk of the V spot (see the diagram on page viii, chapter 3 and chapter 5). It is possible, though not as common, to experience an orgasm in the perineum. In fact, the network of nerves and muscles in this general region creates a pleasure zone, taking in all these areas and an orgasm can be centred anywhere within it. They're all extremely enjoyable, and there's no more merit to one sort than another.

If you become a connoisseur of orgasms, then you'll notice the location of each one and perhaps be able to choose which sort you'd like when you're about to tip over the arousal brink. But if you always have yours in the same place, or are far too absorbed by the passion of the moment to ponder where exactly it's happening, that's absolutely fine too. As ever, just enjoy it.

For many women the optimum sexual high is to

climax with someone they are in love with, as the various chemicals causing the emotion of love merge with those of the orgasm. This produces an all-consuming climax that feels as though mind, body and soul are united in pleasure.

How it happens, physically

Arousal and orgasm are dependent on mind and body working in harmony to integrate our responses to sensual pleasure. This allows a crescendo of feelings to build up in the vaginal and clitoral area and culminates in a cluster of muscle spasms, which cause an explosion of pleasurable sensations. Once the orgasm starts it's impossible to stop it. Much like a sneeze, once triggered, it takes you over with a self-fulfilling imperative and the intense feelings of pleasure are like nothing else.

Our hormonal and neurological systems have a large part to play in the whole pathway of the process, as does muscle tissue, hormone production and the circulatory system. Crucially, the mind comes into it right from our initial willingness to enjoy the pleasure, and our enthusiasm to experience an orgasm smooths out and enables every stage of the journey from the first thought or impulse to it actually happening.

Arousal can be caused by thought or visual or other sensory stimuli and causes an increased flow of blood into and around the vulval area. This swells and reddens the labia and clitoris and relaxes the walls of the vagina, which may secrete extra lubricating fluid.

Other physical effects of arousal and orgasm are:

- an increased heart rate;
- faster and/or deeper breathing;
- flushing of the face, neck and chest;
- swelling and heightened sensitivity of the nipples;
- dilated pupils.

Emotionally, if making love with a partner, you may feel overwhelmed with love for him or her.

As well as allowing and encouraging arousal, the brain has a powerful effect on whether or not arousal translates into climax. Expect to have an orgasm and chances are you will; think you won't and you almost certainly will not. Never is thinking positively more necessary than when making love to yourself or when in the throes of passion with a partner.

Hormones

From the first moment of desire our bodies pitch into a complex chemical reaction that continues right through arousal and helps enable orgasm too. We need certain hormones to feel sexy in the first place and these are principally oestrogen, progesterone and testosterone. Given a sufficient supply of these, the hormones responsible for the exciting feelings of desire, arousal and climax can spring into action.

The main ones are:

- **Phenylethylamine**, the hormone that surges when we have an orgasm is the same hormone that's released when we fall in love (or lust), making us feel dizzy with happiness and on top of the world. It's not surprising we feel euphoric, as it's like an amphetamine in its 'upping' effect. People who are depressed, on the other hand, are generally suffering from too little of it, which can be both a cause and effect of feeling down.
- **Dehydroepiandrosterone**, which also floods the body during arousal and climax, is thought to contribute to a healthy immune system, as well as having other anti-ageing health factors. People who relish their sexuality into old age tend to live longer and I'd hazard a guess that they live happier and healthier lives too.
- Then there's that amazingly good feeling just after orgasm when you feel full of love – for yourself,

your partner or the world. This feel-good hormone is **oxytocin** and is also released in women after childbirth to encourage bonding between mother and child. During foreplay and sex it's produced in both the toucher and the one who is being caressed, particularly during nipple and genital stimulation and intercourse.

- **Endorphins** are well-known for making people feel incredibly good. They're one of the hormones produced during aerobic exercise that give a high to those who dance, run or go to the gym regularly. And they're produced during sex and orgasm. As endorphins are also known to be beneficial for reducing pain, chronic pain sufferers are sometimes advised to make love often. But I wonder if their capacity to relieve pain is due less to their pain-blocking action, which has been described as similar to morphine's, than to the feel-good high they produce in conjunction with the pleasure of sex and orgasm. This not only takes the mind off pain but, in making us feel fantastic, gives us a much more positive attitude to pain and helps us to bear it.

- Finally, there are the sex hormones — most famously **oestrogen** and **testosterone** — which not only are needed for us to become aroused and climax, but whose production increases in the process.

Final ingredients for the alchemy of arousal and orgasm

If hormones and muscles and the wish to enjoy sexual pleasure were all that were needed, we'd all be having great orgasmic sex effortlessly on a daily basis. But three more ingredients are needed to mobilise the alchemy and enable it to transform the elements into easy, pleasurable sexual fulfilment.

They are:

1. **Discovery of the techniques that work for you.** In the sections on becoming orgasmic by yourself and with a partner, I give the best techniques I've found that work for most people. Have fun finding which ones most appeal to you, turn you on the best and easily take you over the brink into orgasm. We're all different and the slightest nuance of tone or touch in any aspect of eroticism could be the catalyst that enables arousal and orgasm for you. Exploring possibilities when you're fully relaxed and not in a rush is a fabulous experience.
2. **Practice.** Throughout this book, there are references to the enabling power of practice and habit. It isn't

just that practice enables ability, improves skills in becoming and being aroused and being orgasmic; practice has another subtler but perhaps even more powerful effect: making love often or at least reasonably regularly conditions us physiologically to doing so on an ongoing basis.

Physically, the chemicals associated with sexual pleasure flow more generously when we make love frequently and regularly. It seems that the hormone-releasing centres get into the habit of producing, and when you make love regularly, they boost their numbers in anticipation of your next session.

This works mentally, too: if you know you're likely to make love that night, for example, and enjoy anticipating the sensations every now and then throughout the day, you'll trigger a steady flow of the hormones that enable arousal and pleasure. By the time you do make love, you'll find you get turned on really easily with your senses already awake to stimulation and primed to take you straight into the arousal curve and along into orgasm.

All in all, the old adage 'the more you do it, the more you can do it' is particularly true for enjoying satisfying, orgasmic sex and a vibrant sexual vitality.

3. **Positive thinking.** If you think you'll have an orgasm, you probably will. If you get into the habit of thinking of yourself as an ultra-feminine, sexy woman who is comfortable with her sexuality and enjoys sex often, that's exactly who you will be.

Arousal and the ecstasy of orgasm are often described as feeling magically good so no matter how many medical discoveries prove it's a chemical reaction, or how many new techniques enhance our skills, it will always feel electrifying. That's the wonder of great sex.

The importance of orgasm in our lives

Is it essential for us to have orgasms? Well, we can certainly exist without them and many women who don't have orgasms don't miss them in any way. So, no, they are not necessarily essential to our emotional or physical health, or our fulfilment and our happiness generally.

But having said that, many women, whether or not they are orgasmic, do feel orgasms are an intrinsic part of well-being and believe that, if they don't have them, they are missing out on a vital element. With only one exception, the women I discussed this with who are currently not orgasmic all said they would like to be able to enjoy effortless, supremely pleasurable arousal and climax.

What is an Orgasm?

There's certainly a lot to be said for being easily orgasmic. Apart from the obvious physical pleasure, it does wonders for our self-confidence. Knowing you can give yourself such a deep treat of pleasure whenever you wish gives you a sense of being good to yourself and at one with your femininity, sexuality and sensuality. It's a deep source of personal satisfaction.

If you're in a relationship, being orgasmic is great for that too. When you've made love and climaxed, you feel full of love towards your partner and both cherished and cherishing. And just as it's a great feeling for you when he has an orgasm, so it is for him when you do. It also improves casual sex tremendously if you are able to have an orgasm easily – with a casual partner you're less likely to have the benefit of a thoughtful, 'let's take our time' mutual attitude so if you can adapt your arousal curve and orgasm to the pace of the encounter, it will be more satisfying all round.

Giving and receiving pleasure draws a couple emotionally close. The mixed feeling of surrender as you have an orgasm because of your partner's lovemaking, and of the power you feel as he has one because of yours, is deliciously pleasant and bonding.

I feel more macho when she comes: David's story

I love it when Jess gets aroused and especially when she comes. It makes me feel strong and macho – powerful, I suppose. And it makes me feel very tender and loving towards her. I'm afraid I do tend to go off to sleep straight after we've made love, but even the next morning it will still be very much on our minds that we both came and we'll be very loving and warm with each other. It makes you feel very close, very together.

Orgasm can be a spiritual experience: Sophie's story

Sometimes we feel as if we connect in another dimension as well as the obvious physical and emotional one. We're not religious but my partner and I believe there is much more to our reality than has yet been discovered. I'm sure we have souls and when we make love orgasmically, it's as though time stops for a moment of shared beauty and union. It sounds such a cliché but that's how it is.

The exercise we experience during sex is good for our body tone and circulation and the range of feel-good hormones that are released during arousal and climax are great for the mind too. While orgasm isn't an essential element of good health, it can be a huge benefit.

Last but not least, we should not dismiss the fact that we have a monthly cycle, and though fertile for just a few days mid-term and most easily aroused then, we can experience desire and feel sexy at any time of the month. We are designed to be orgasmic – it's natural so typically it feels good when we are.

Casual sex has improved: Lou's story

Now that I usually climax easily and quickly, sex with someone new is much better. I used to wonder why I bothered having casual sex because I didn't orgasm unless they were willing to take lots of time and were really good lovers – and that hardly ever happened. These days I'm much less reliant on a partner's technique, knowing that I can guide them into a position and tempo that will turn me on. My own pleasure is in my control and it's rare that I don't have an orgasm.

Desire and arousal

In the usual way of things, orgasm is preceded by arousal and desire. Desire can be sparked by a compelling physical urge to have sex or simply the thought that it would be a good idea, followed by an 'Okay, let's do it' decision. Given your go-ahead (and sometimes without it) this leads to arousal — an increased blood flow to the genitals, and often to the nipples and lips as well, and the heightened sensitivity of nerve endings of your whole body.

The whole process can take as little as a minute or two (this is very rare) to about 20 minutes or more (this is more likely) and can be prolonged for hours. Generally, quickie orgasms are not as powerful as those that have a longer build-up, probably because with the speed of the climax being mind-driven, the genitals haven't had a chance to completely engorge, nor have the nerve endings reached their full sensitivity. If you've never spent longer than a few minutes in arousal and you've never had an orgasm, taking more time to let desire build could be the orgasmic answer.

We usually start to be beguiled by our awakening sexual feelings around puberty and during our teenage years. Often our first teenage crush involves a celebrity heart-throb like a musician or an actor. Even now, if I hear a record that takes me back to that exciting decade of my life, it brings up those first passions in all their uncon-summated innocence and safety.

Adoration of romantic idols is good preparation and practice in our sexual epiphany before we're ready for the real thing. Then, through the course of a few friendships, as we enjoy romance and petting we learn more about our feelings of desire and arousal and get used to calling them up, smoothing them down or even ignoring them, as appropriate for the situation. We learn the difference between lust and being in love, and between being in love and loving in a deeper, potentially lasting way. Then, if all goes to plan, we exist happily for the rest of our lives with desire and arousal as a consistent part of our sex drive.

Of course life – and our sex drive – is rarely perfect. Maybe you were discouraged from early infatuations with pop stars, or were scared or disinterested in your emerging sexual feelings and suppressed them by throwing yourself into studies or sports. Or perhaps your parents made you feel sex was bad and shameful.

Another possible scenario is that your sexual development went well but somewhere along the line it was damaged by a partner or by something that happened in your life that changed your perception and experience of sex. Our sex drive is prone to changing, sometimes dramatically, at various stages of our lives. As you age, you may find your body is less easily aroused into wanting sex than your mind, or perhaps both give up on sex. If so, the fact that you're reading this suggests that your mind is not so ready to give it up; after all, desire, arousal and satisfaction are all intensely pleasurable and are good for our individual happiness and our relationships (if we're in one).

Fortunately, all is not lost if desire and arousal do fade or disappear — it is definitely possible to bring them back to life again. With a combination of the advice in this book and your gut feeling you can work out the possible reasons for losing desire or intensity of arousal, and passionately plan to bring them back. Sure, it may not be the same as it used to be, as we are constantly changing throughout our lives, but your sexuality can, if you wish, stay with you. Sexuality is not governed by your partner or lack of a partner, hormones or chemicals — it's largely dependent on your mindset.

I went off sex: Brenda's story

I had a history of going off sex and my partners. In the early stages of the relationship I'd fancy them like mad, and this could last from a couple of months to even a few years. Then, like a light switching off, the attraction would be gone and either I'd finish with them or they'd dump me because they were fed up with me refusing sex. I often used to think, 'If I met someone as gorgeous as Johnny Depp, I'd desire them forever.' But then I happened to see Johnny Depp in a new film one day and to my disappointment he did nothing for me. It was then when I realised my previous desire had little to do with his looks and that beauty in itself does not mean that someone is sexy – it's character that turns me on.

From then on I didn't go out with anyone until I met a man whose mind rather than looks excited and interested me. My relationship with Doug has been the best, longest-lasting one I've ever had – but it almost hit the deck a couple of years ago when I had to have a hysterectomy. I hadn't gone off him – Doug was as charismatic for me as ever – it was simply that my mind and body were affected by unsettled hormones and had stopped prompting desire. Once again, I was off sex and not having orgasms. Sex meant a lot to us, and so, following your advice, whenever it seemed apt for me, I gradually practised getting physically fit again and cajoling my mind back to feeling sexy too. Although the input had to be mine essentially, Doug helped a lot by not pressuring me, and by willingly giving me wonderful massages or long stroking sessions that brought back my capacity for sensual pleasure. In time this morphed into sexual desire and arousal, and once they were back, so were my orgasms.

Hormones are powerful, for sure, but our minds are more powerful and can often override any hormonal or physical lack.

Would Viagra help?

Current thinking is that the reason for Viagra and similar drugs not working so well on women is because arousal and desire are not always linked like they are for men. While in our youthful years a purely physical urge is often enough to prompt desire and can rush us along the arousal curve, as we mature, the majority of women find that mind plays a very important part in turning us on. However, anything that helps physically is worth consideration, so it will be interesting to follow studies on any new drugs and therapies.

It's good to remember that it's you who holds the keys to arousal in your own mind, so think about what makes you feel sexy, drives desire and intensifies arousal. Bring the equation into your life physically and equally vividly in your mind and orgasm will follow.

Making time, taking time

When we're young and discovering sexual pleasure, we're fascinated with it and want a lot of it. We don't need to make time for it — we're already thinking about it and doing it as often as possible, naturally and spontaneously. Effort? No way!

The same goes for new relationships; at any time in our lives they're exciting — the attraction and desire utterly compelling — so however busy our schedules, however great our responsibilities, we make time and take time.

And for some the excitement and novelty of youthful or new relationship sex is orgasmic. But for many it makes for sex that's too quick or even just too passionate to learn how to have orgasms. So, if this has been your scenario of sex so far, you could have had a healthily good sex drive and a lot of pleasure, but missed out on orgasms.

For those who were orgasmic but aren't now, it's probable that once past early or new affair fascination, they found sexual pleasure and climax became less and less spontaneous, and other pastimes and commitments and simple lack of energy gained ground until sexual interest and orgasms declined, and maybe stopped completely.

I've counselled so many women who weren't or were hardly ever making love, yet bemoaned the fact and complained about being anorgasmic. Often, they'll blame it on waning desire, or a reduced capacity for arousal. Some think they need to be in love to enjoy great sex, and blame their anorgasmia on the fact that they're not.

If any of these scenarios apply to you, take heart. Yes, you can get the magic of sexual pleasure back, and yes, you can become orgasmic or, if you used to be, regain the knack.

The key is acknowledging the truth that for women, and many men, spontaneity often evaporates once the excitement phase of novelty and early attraction passes. Like any activity, however much we enjoy it, we have to choose to do it. Like most skills, the more we practise, the easier and more satisfying it becomes to do and to make it a regular habit.

Make the commitment to have sex with yourself or with a partner at least once a week. The point is to practise and practise and practise until orgasms start to come and eventually you can give yourself one whenever you want.

What is an Orgasm?

No time? Make time. Too stressed? Tell yourself sex will relax you (it will). Too tired? Remember that once pleasure begins, you'll enjoy it, no matter how tired you are (you will). Know that you'll sleep blissfully well (you will). Elbow the sessions into your diary, however busy you are. This is important to you, deeply important – you wouldn't be reading this book if it weren't. Make time and take time to enjoy yourself, your sexual self, and once you know how, give yourself the joy of an orgasm.

Chapter 2

Loving Yourself, Loving Your Body

Liking and being at peace with ourselves helps us to accept and enjoy our sexuality. There's nothing like a confident approach to life and high self-esteem to encourage a positive, relaxed expectation of a satisfying sex life and contentment with your sexuality. If you think you're sexy, you *are* sexy, and feeling really bubbly and vibrant and exuberantly in love with life is a great aphrodisiac.

What does this have to do with me not having orgasms?

It may be a crucial factor. If your self-esteem or self-confidence is low, it could be causing a loop of thinking that speaks to you consciously or unconsciously when you're having sex, saying, 'You won't have an orgasm,' or,

'You're hopeless; you're a failure.' This immediately sends a message to your neurological system that orgasm isn't going to happen and it won't, because you've effectively programmed it not to.

A blow to self-esteem: Jay's story

I used to be orgasmic, but when I lost my previous job, the sense of failure permeated every aspect of my life, including my sex drive. What should have given me a release from the gloom deepened it even more because I couldn't get into the spirit of it. I was apathetic about making love and couldn't even be bothered to masturbate – I'd do it for a couple of minutes and think, 'It's no good; I'm not going to enjoy it and there's no way I'll have an orgasm so what's the point.' Gradually, working with a cognitive behaviour counsellor, I learnt to use affirmations and reasoning to lift me out of the blues and by expecting to enjoy sex again and be orgasmic, I made it happen. I have recurrent down times but I know what to do now and refuse to let it affect my sex life – it's a precious part of my self-esteem and love of life and I'm looking after it from now on, whatever happens.

With high self-esteem and self-confidence you'll be able to practise saying to yourself, 'I'm an orgasmic woman and I love the pleasures of sex,' giving your whole sexual system the go-ahead to enjoy the arousal curve right up to the brink of orgasm and all the way over it, to the ecstasy.

Building self-esteem

If you suffer from low self-esteem, you're unlikely to reach your full potential in life, and it will also affect your enthusiasm for sex and capacity for pleasure, including climaxing.

It's easy to blame our self-esteem, however much of it we have or lack, on our parents – and there's no doubt about it, they usually shape it. Often children who suffer from low self-esteem continue to as adults.

Whatever the reasons, if you don't think enough of yourself and your abilities, it's important to remember you can rise above or circumvent them, build a healthy, feel-good level of self-esteem and confidence, and maintain it forever.

You are at the controls of your being, your attitude and your life. No one else can force your sense of self-worth away from you if you believe in yourself. That belief is an attitude you choose, every day of your life. Start now – you are a wonderful person, a wonderful, orgasmic person.

Begin nurturing your self-esteem today with a change of attitude. If only it were that simple, you're probably thinking. But I promise you, it really is. That's not to say you'll wave a magic wand and immediately start to think positive about yourself. It will take a lot of ongoing practice but you do have the courage and the ability – as testified by the fact you're reading this book.

You can raise your self-esteem swiftly in three ways – affirmation, reason and behaviour. They work best hand-in-hand.

How to have good self-esteem

First of all, you need to quash your inner critic. Give yourself a daily mantra, such as: 'Today I am going to think of myself as a nice person.'

By all means substitute a word of your choosing if you're not happy with 'nice' because you think it's boring or goody-two-shoes. It could, for instance, be 'great' or 'lovable' or 'special' – all of which you are. All I ask is that it's 100 per cent positive.

Use it every day, first thing when you wake up and any time you're putting yourself down or you become aware that someone else is. Using it not only reminds you that you are a good person, it will actually change your aura, body language and behaviour and affect those around you positively too.

Sceptical? Many people are initially and I completely understand. But try it and you will see for yourself that it has an extraordinary effect. See my books *Think Love* and *Free Your Life From Fear* for more help with this.

The effect you want most in the context of this book is for your self-esteem to flourish so that your sexual enjoyment will reach its full potential.

Reason and logic

If something's recently dented your self-esteem or it's habitually low after years of conditioning, you'll need to create or reinforce a sound foundation for your affirmation that you're a nice and valuable person.

Reason and logic are the tools for this and if used with scrupulous honesty and good sense, they will open your eyes to all the positive elements of your character, and also nurture you as you mature towards your full potential.

Who are you?

A good starting point to feeling good is to make a list of all your positive attributes. I do this every few weeks just to 'top-up'. Put down anything that comes to mind and include things you're good at as well as character traits.

If your self-esteem and self-image are very low, you may struggle, so ask a good friend to help out. Don't be scared of doing this – your friends and family will love thinking of the things they admire or like about you.

Ask a friend for help: Karen's story

I had to ask a friend to give me a reference to support my application for a course I wanted to go on. I was surprised by the attributes she mentioned, which included a couple of things that I wouldn't have even thought applied to me. It gave me a huge boost and the incentive to keep paying attention to my self-esteem and keep it healthy.

Use this foundation of positive attributes to reason with yourself if ever your self-confidence takes a knock. Register what you're feeling and, once acknowledged, start thinking yourself back into balance again. For instance, if you are criticised, take the points made onboard and weigh them to see what you can do to improve if necessary, and more importantly, to remember that criticism need never sink you – you can use it, instead, as a tool to help you think the issue through and grow from it. Thus, whatever happens to us in life is a part of our maturing process — an opportunity to learn about ourselves and keep developing.

Remind yourself, whenever your confidence takes a knock, of your abilities and your achievements, your best character traits — being kind, loving, supportive to others, a good leader or team member — whatever springs to mind.

Be friends with yourself

When you have a really good friend — one who you trust, like and enjoy being with, one you can be totally honest with, you don't care what they look like — you just love them.

Treat yourself like a cherished friend. Listen to your thoughts, your body and your soul. Take time to pay attention like this for it is the way you will learn more and more about yourself and the best path for you.

Be your own best friend: Cheryl's story

I often talk to myself — out loud sometimes, if I'm alone — to help me work things out and to give myself a sense of support. It sounds dippy but it helps to ground me, think things through and make decisions. I'll give myself a mental hug if I'm feeling down, and suggest ways to recover. I've some good friends, two of whom I'm very close to and who know me very well indeed, but they can't always be there for me, whereas I can be my own full-time best friend.

It's helped me sexually too – if ever there's been a problem, I help myself work out what my partner or I can do. So when I became unable to climax, I didn't pretend it wasn't happening or that it didn't matter – I felt the worry and said to myself it was probably just a phase. But it turned out it wasn't – it went on and on and then it was as though my body said to me, 'For goodness sake, do something about this – we're missing out!' So I found a counsellor and set about bringing back my ability to have orgasms. Although my friends are wonderful, I couldn't have talked to my friends about it as I would have been embarrassed, and anyway, they probably would have been at a loss as to what advice to give me. I knew deep down I needed help and sought it. It felt good in every way to be so constructive and, in just a few weeks, be able to correct what my counsellor called the 'tripped switch' and start being orgasmic again. I couldn't have done it without the loving communication between my mind, body and soul.

Like yourself, value yourself, love yourself, be your own best friend. It's all part of being orgasmic.

Love yourself

Isn't it a bit narcissistic to love yourself? Not at all — if you love yourself, you'll be able to love others more. Love yourself and you'll be most of the way to being happy with your sexuality, sensuality and orgasmability. Love yourself and you'll welcome and accept your loved ones' love and, in so doing, attract it.

It's all a circle, but I put self-esteem first in this section because developing it is straightforward. Once you think positively about yourself, it's much easier to love yourself. Loving is often not spontaneous but an emotion we choose to feel. Through building your self-esteem dissolves a 'What's to love about me?' mindset and enables you to see the myriad lovable things about you.

Practise now making the shift to positively, warmly, lovingly loving yourself. Look in the mirror, smile warmly and say, 'I love you' to yourself. If ever you're hurt in some way or a bit down, give yourself a big mental hug. Or take yourself back to being a little girl in the snug security of your mum's arms. You are still that little girl. You are very, very lovable but these days love for yourself starts with you.

Loving yourself is often a key to being orgasmic, as if you don't or feel you shouldn't, you may be sabotaging your ability to climax by programming your mind and body connection to not accept the pleasure.

Orgasm is an amazing, beautiful gift we give to ourselves. The best lover in the world won't be able to help you have or 'give' you an orgasm if your mind is in some way set against it. When you love yourself, you tacitly say 'yes' to the joy of orgasm.

Self-love may also enable you to truly love your partner instead of confusing it with neediness or greediness. Such negative reasons don't work for orgasm – in fact, they won't bring happiness in any aspect of your life. The more you snatch at sexual pleasure and try to force orgasm, the less likely it is to happen. On the other hand, if you relax into love for love's sake – unconditional, warm, sincere love – you'll undoubtedly open the gates for pleasure and joy of all kinds, including orgasm.

Loving your body

If someone wants to make love to you, rest assured they think you are beautiful whether you are stereotypically beautiful or not. The sexiest thing for your partner is your willingness to forget what you look like and abandon yourself to the pleasure you're sharing. Yes, men tend to be more visually turned on than women so they'll love to look at you. But more than anything they want, as soon as possible, to be close up against you, feeling your body against theirs, smelling you, tasting you, loving you and being loved by you. So lose your self-consciousness – it won't help your love life one bit and is unnecessary once you accept that he adores making love to you and that the last thing he'll do is look at you critically when you're having a great time.

By all means relish the beauty of your bodies as you move together – but use it as an aphrodisiac, never critically or to deflect your attention from the pleasures of making love.

Sex just gets better with age: Judy's story

When I was young, I was a model and I knew my body was stunning. But in a way it detracted from my enjoyment of sex as I was so anxious to show it off to its best effect that I spent more time positioning and posturing than letting go and having a good time. I quite liked sex but never had an orgasm because I was far too uptight. Then thankfully I noticed that lovers weren't interested in looking at me in awe and admiring me – or my designer underwear, come to that – they wanted to cuddle and hug and connect with me. So I stopped thinking about what I looked like and loosened up. Suddenly, I realised how fantastic sex could be – earthy, schmoozy, a complete turn-on – and one day I had this incredible orgasm, which had me crying and laughing with surprise and happiness. Thank goodness I made the discovery that bodies feel good in bed and looks don't matter at all, because I realise now that while my figure's not what it was, my partner thinks the world of me and we have an orgasmic time in bed.

Being happy to be you

Happiness and contentment enable and enhance our ability to have and fully enjoy a healthy sex drive along with sexual pleasure and orgasms. Yes, we *can* be sexy and orgasmic when we're unhappy and discontented. In the early days of a relationship the excitement may blow away or at least counteract any depression, apathy or frustration which had been causing low libido or difficulty climaxing. But more often than not, whether you're single or in a long-term relationship, negativity lowers sex drive and, along with it, the ability to have orgasms.

Happiness can be made or disrupted by many different things. If you are dissatisfied, check out whichever sections of this book you sense may be apt for your happiness needs. For instance, look at raising your self-esteem, or perhaps some relatively straightforward practical steps are needed to change an aspect of your life that's sabotaging any chance of contentment just now. If you're often over-pressured and stressed, for instance, creating a good work-life balance could revolutionise your emotional and physical energy and transform your libido, sensuality and orgasmability.

What if there's not much to like? Then change yourself!

Certainly, most of us will at some time or several times in our lives notice that we're not currently behaving in a particularly likeable or applaudable way. It's easy to be influenced by the callousness of others, for example, and to learn to get in first with the arrows of negativity, cutting remarks or unkind actions. When we behave uncaringly or, worse, downright spitefully, it, without fail, rebounds on us. If you actively cause other people to dislike or fear you, you will dislike and fear yourself. That will have a knock-on effect on any relationships – somewhere deep down you'll feel you don't deserve a partner's love or to have a warm, enjoyable, orgasmic sex life. It's the same if you're habitually dishonest – financially or in just about any way. Lies and deception weave a sticky web around happiness and sooner or later stand to sabotage your innate sexiness too.

If this is ringing bells with you, well done for being honest enough to admit it. Now you have the chance to make it up to anyone you've intentionally hurt and start from now onwards being kind, warm and positive – in other words treating everyone you meet as a human being who, even if he or she has a veneer of success and confidence, is every bit as vulnerable and fragile as you.

It may sound sugary and corny to recommend being nice but on the whole it makes others feel good – and you too. The only people who won't like the new positive, warm you are those who are so entrenched in their cynicism that they can't stand goodness. But they've been adversely affecting your self-esteem for far too long – don't let them influence your behaviour any more.

When you behave warmly and kindly to others, you'll feel good about yourself and learn to like yourself, enabling a healthy self-esteem, which in turn helps to enable confident sensuality and sexuality.

And change your life

Similarly, if your self-esteem is low because you're dissatisfied with any practical aspect of your life, over the next few weeks or months appraise what you've achieved and where you are now. Start thinking about where you would like to be in, say, two years' time and what you would like to achieve by then and beyond. This could have to do with your career progression or with your home life. Perhaps you will want to make plans and begin to put them into action. Alternatively, the appraisal may be very useful in helping you realise that actually your life is pretty good just as it is: often other people's ambitions, or all the stuff we see in the media about super-rich celebrities, can make us feel dissatisfied with what we've got, when, in fact, what we've got is fine in its own right. Fantastic looks and riches do not make us happy – happiness is an attitude, a take on life that sees the good all around us, putting the negative side into perspective, and that helps us relish our myriad comforts and blessings, our vitality and passion, our joy in life. Take charge of your life and your attitude to your life. It will increase your sexiness and your orgasmability!

Building high self-esteem and confidence

- Review your present situation regularly. If you feel you are trapped or have little control over your situation, consider how you can start taking charge of your path and make improvements. Even if you can't change certain circumstances, you can find ways to improve the quality of your life by changing your attitude or seeking out and enlisting a better support network.
- Aim to improve the balance between the negative influences and the things that enhance your life.
- Don't be a victim. Remember that you have tremendous personal power.
- See the good all around you and be glad for it. Most of being fortunate is feeling fortunate – and counting your blessings is a great way to instantly boost your self-esteem.
- Make a list of things to do today, this week, by the end of the month and year as a useful way to focus your mind. As you tick things off or make progress towards a long-term goal the

satisfaction will be immense. Don't fret if you don't do everything on the short-term lists — put them on your new ones and prioritise them. Completion is preceded by aim, focus, perseverance and the process from start to finish feels good and boosts self-esteem.

- Consider people and places with whom and where you feel safe and spend some time there as often as possible. Such havens help us balance the challenges of life, help us feel lovable and foster happiness.

- Be interested in yourself — the way you've developed and why and the kind of person you are. We are all multifaceted and being aware of our complexity without denying less pleasant elements helps us accept ourselves, warts and all, and enables us to grow in wisdom and goodness. Of course you're not perfect — but, hey, you're doing all right! No matter what has happened to you in the past and however you have behaved to others or they to you, you are now focused on living well, integrating the various elements of your personality and valuing yourself fully as well as those you love.

- We all experience a mixture of emotions — positive ones like love, kindness, generosity, humour and tolerance, and negative ones like dislike, jealousy, bitterness, shame and spite. Trying to force the negative ones underground or pretending they don't exist puts you into a state of denial, which will undermine your self-esteem and confidence because it means you're living a lie. Feeling you're a horrible person is no more helpful — it just leads to depression. It's best to acknowledge that you, like everyone else, sometimes have bad feelings and thoughts but remind yourself that you are free to choose not to dwell on them.

- Drop your negative baggage. You don't have to carry a load of it around with you!

- Play, laugh and notice the funny things and absurdities of the day.

Remember that when you make love to yourself or with a partner, the better you feel about yourself, the better and more orgasmic the lovemaking will be.

Chapter 3

How to Have an Orgasm on Your Own

It's liberating to know you are not dependent on a partner to feel sexy and sensual and to know that whenever you choose you can pleasure yourself all the way to climax. It's also good to know that if you know your own body – what turns you on and makes you orgasmic – then sex with a partner will only get better.

It saddens me that some women think it's wrong to enjoy their sexuality alone. It's utterly natural for us to enjoy our own bodies and I can think of no reason not to appreciate the pleasure we can give ourselves. So go for it. You have nothing to lose by learning to give yourself orgasms and everything to gain.

Choosing a good place
Where do you need to be to give yourself sexual pleasure

that includes orgasm? Somewhere where you are alone and where you've no fear of being interrupted. Your home is the obvious choice until you're experienced and confident in bringing yourself to orgasm, as it's essential that you're in a place where you can utterly relax. When you know exactly how it works for you and can easily put your preferences of touch into practice, an element of excitement can be used to trigger orgasm, but that's some way ahead. For now, choose a place where you're physically comfortable and where you're sure no one is going to disturb you – if possible, somewhere where you can lock the door. Better still, choose a time when you're completely alone in your home and you can safely anticipate solitude for at least half an hour.

Let's look at the possible locations:

- **The bedroom** – There are so many advantages to choosing the bedroom: a comfortable bed where you can move about as much as you want with no hard surfaces or edges to hurt yourself; a sense of freedom to do as you want and, knowing that even if you don't have a lock on the door, it's normally understood that if the door is shut, your bedroom is a private place and no one will enter without asking.

- The bathroom – This has several advantages; for one thing, there's probably a lock on the door so you can be sure no one's going to come bursting in.

  Pleasuring yourself in a warm bath relaxes you and some women find the feel of the water around them, particularly if pleasantly scented, is sensuous in itself and very conducive to arousal. There's no doubt about it, a warm bath is a great place to masturbate. But there are several disadvantages as far as orgasm is concerned – baths tend to be quite hard so it's not that comfortable to move about in them; most baths aren't big enough for you to really stretch out your legs; and, you tend to get too hot for comfort, and while a bit of heat is orgasmic, too much is not. Again, when you're confidently orgasmic, you may find you can climax in the bath and that's fine, but even the most experienced women tend to use a warm bath for a prelude of self-pleasure and go for the finale somewhere else.

  Another potentially very erotic and orgasmic possibility is in the bath or shower, to direct the shower hose so that the warm water streams down over your clitoris. (Make sure not to direct it up towards your vulva, though, as it has been suggested that water can be forced into the urethra this way, and can cause infection.)

- **The living room** — The comfort of a sofa you can relax and stretch out in is good in theory. And a rug in front of a fire, though something of a cliché for relationship sex, can be a good place to pleasure yourself too, as long as it's thick enough to cushion you from the hard floor. But once more there is a disadvantage: I and many of the women I've talked to find that the living room is a public place, off-putting for such a private and personal pastime, even if there's no one else in the house. Even those women I talked to who enjoy having an orgasm in their living area agreed that for first-time orgasm it wasn't the best idea.

So whether you're going for your first orgasm ever or renewing your ability to be easily orgasmic when you wish, I recommend you choose your bedroom and your bed.

If you're thinking that this is obvious stuff, then just skip the sections until you come to something that may make a difference to you becoming orgasmic. Orgasm is such a finely tuned response for each of us that the tiniest thing can stop us having one. Finding the block, on the other hand, and making sure it can't snarl things up again, can open the way to what many think is one of the most mind-blowing sensations we

can have — so it's worth looking at anything and everything that's going to make it easier.

Setting the mood

The room should be somewhere where you can easily
relax. You should be able to feel content just being there
and good about yourself, too — the best starting points
to being orgasmic. So make sure the room is inviting and
that you like the look of it. However much space, make
it an inspiring and relaxing place to be and orgasms will
come more easily. Also, as every orgasm is in a sense a
luxury we treat ourselves to, surroundings we love accen-
tuate that sense and enhance sensuality and arousal.

If you like to have a glass of wine and know it makes
you feel sexy or less inhibited, by all means, do. Music you
love can also help you get in the mood for sexual pleasure, and scented candles or your own favourite perfume
all add to the erotic ambience.

Fantasies can be very erotic too. (See Complement
arousal with fantasy on page 76 for more on this.)

The straightforward way to give yourself an orgasm

This is the sure-fire technique to arouse yourself and
open the way to being orgasmic. It even works if you

have no preliminary physical urge for sex. For example, if you happen to be going through a hormonal or stressful phase of your life when desire for sexual pleasure has deserted you, this way will swiftly spark your interest and put you on the arousal path to a good climax.

Once you've practised the technique and are thoroughly relaxed with it, do try out other ways if you wish. It's fun finding out what works best for you and to personalise your favourite ways to give yourself an orgasm.

It may surprise you, if you've already taken a look first at the section on being orgasmic in a relationship, that for your first and future orgasms on your own I recommend going straight into genital touch – which is the opposite of my advice for being orgasmic with a partner. When two people make love, it's usually sexiest and most successful for her when they build arousal via all the other erogenous zones as I explain in detail. With a partner, genital touch early in a lovemaking session doesn't work so well because we women like, and usually need, to be seduced or to have intimacy reaffirmed before we go genital, and that takes a while.

But when you're pleasuring yourself, it's a different matter –you don't need to be persuaded and/or relaxed because you're already naturally familiar and intimate with yourself. Most of all, you know you've decided to give yourself the enjoyment of an orgasm and the easiest way to become sexually aroused, on your own, is to gently pleasure your clitoris and surrounding area straight off.

What's the best position?

At first – and until you master becoming orgasmic – I recommend lying flat on your back with your head resting on a soft pillow. Your legs should be slightly apart and either stretched out or with your knees drawn up towards you and your feet resting flat on the bed. In this position you're perfectly stable so you don't have to think about anything other than touch and feel, and you can easily rock yourself, pivot your pelvis and arch your back.

If, like some women, you feel self-conscious to be, as one of my clients put it, 'too blatantly spread out', try lying on your side, or sitting in a comfortable chair where you can slip your bum forwards when you want to arch your pelvis against your hand. It helps if the chair has a firm back for support.

If you're not sure which most appeals, another good option is a combination of elements of two or all of these suggestions. You could start off by sitting on the edge of the bed with your feet on the floor, for instance, then move right on to the bed and lie on your side and then, as excitement grows, make another half turn on to your back. With practice, you'll soon find the position or variety of positions that works best for you.

The touch technique

Your own hand is simply the best possible means to make love to yourself. By caressing yourself with the direct, immediate touch of your hand, you are absolutely clear on what you are doing and at the same time wherever you are touching yourself – your clitoris, V spot, wherever – you'll obviously feel it and the nerve endings there will form a kind of dialogue with those in your fingers. Later, vibrators and other sex toys can be fun to use and expand your portfolio of pleasure. For now, as you learn about your unique way of experiencing pleasure while you masturbate, using your hand is by far the best way. The direct contact is totally natural, ultra-sensitive, gives the best feedback and, in my opinion, the best orgasms.

The first time you try this technique I would recommend that you don't use fantasy – this will help you stay focused on the feel of touch on your clitoral and vulval area and let it intensify into a crescendo that is natural to you.

Step 1: Liberally apply some lubricant to the whole of your vulva, starting at and around the clitoris and including the labia and spreading it right down to and around the opening of your vagina. You want to be nice and silky-slippery so there's no chance of sore friction.

Step 2: Before you even start to use your hand you should test on various parts of your body what your mouth, tongue and moist lips feel like as they touch, kiss and caress your skin, pressing, stroking and licking. It feels and tastes good, doesn't it? The sensations you enjoy the most are what you are aiming to replicate when you use your fingers.

Step 3: Use the hand that feels most apt – probably your right hand if you're right-handed. Later it can be interesting to use your other hand or both sets of fingers to make it feel like someone else is touching you, but for now, let's focus on one hand and two fingers as you want to be aware of how the whole area feels to your fingers, and how your fingertips feel.

Step 4: Now practise your touch, but not genitally just yet. Place the tip of your first finger on the back of your other hand and keeping it in that exact place (ie without rubbing from side to side across the skin) gently move the skin over the tissues beneath. The skin on the back of the hand or, for another example, on the underside of our wrists, tends to be quite loose and you'll probably find you can move the skin in this way without moving what's underneath. In other areas, like further up your arm, you'll find the same movement will move the flesh underneath at the same time. Get it as close as you can to the feeling of your mouth and remember how it feels to the fingertips too, so you can then transfer it to your vulva and imagine the sensations are not being produced by your fingers, but by someone giving you oral sex.

Which do you prefer? The sensations when you acknowledge they're being made by you with your fingertips? Or the sensations when you forget your hands are responsible and imagine they are being produced by someone else's mouth? Either is absolutely fine – go with whichever you prefer or, as many women like, sometimes one, and sometimes the other.

Try different pressures. What feels good? Very light or slightly firmer? Perhaps sometimes much firmer? Alternate the pressure and the tempo. Apply this kind of touch, in as many ways, to lots of places on your body – it's delicious just about everywhere. Which are your favourite places? Your temples maybe? Your arms? Or perhaps your feet? It's interesting that the most popular massages are back, feet, head and neck so for many people, these are our top-most non-genital sensuous zones.

As you discover your most sensual places, your entire skin will start to feel alert – waiting and hoping for attention.

This practice of familiarising yourself with your pleasure zones – perhaps the skin over all your body, perhaps a few specific places that you love best – will soon make you an expert in touch both of your whole body and of your orgasmic touch too.

Step 5: Using the tips of your first and second fingers, feel your clitoris through its covering hood, gently stroking or pressing as you move the skin beneath it in small circles. Don't ever rub your clitoris, as even when protected by its hood it is ultra-sensitive and responds better to the gentlest whisper of touch through to firmer (but still gentle) pressure. Rubbing not only doesn't feel as good, it is likely to cause discomfort and put you off the whole idea. The little hood, too, though much more robust than the tissues of the clitoris it protects, is only a layer of skin and needs to be gently treated.

Step 6: Register how your touch feels. How does each kind of touch, such as pressing, circling or stroking feel? How does it feel to your fingertips?

At first, most women find that until sensitivity increases as the clitoris and surrounding area are charged with the increased blood flow to the area, the feeling receptors respond best to a rhythmic pressing touch combined or alternating with a small circulating fingertip movement.

Step 7: Touching yourself in the way you've practised, feel your clitoris through its covering – that is, from just above it – then move upwards again, focusing on the clitoral shaft between your clitoris and the place where your vulva begins. Now explore the pubic bone that meets it, still pressing gently and rhythmically.

Step 8: Next, explore the outer labia, taking in the area on both sides between your vulva and the top of each leg. Then, skirting the entrance to your vagina, feel your perineum gently and then slide your hand underneath and around the cheeks of your bottom. Notice when your buttocks are gently massaged they may be a surprisingly erogenous zone.

Step 9: Now bring your fingertips back to your vulva and travel up the inner lips to come back to your clitoris. Try touching it directly now. If you find this stimulating, make sure you're still well lubricated (if not apply more) and let your fingers press or stroke this sensitive place, softly, caressingly, firmly or alternating — whichever you prefer.

If, like many women, you find direct clitoral touch too intense, go back to the comfort and luxury of the less sensitive but more sensual covering above and around it. The uncovered tip of the clitoris is sometimes compared to the glans of a penis; in a circumcised man it loses the natural intense sensitivity but when it is protected by his foreskin, as the clitoris is by its hood, it usually remains too sensitive for much, if any, direct manual stimulation and moving the foreskin over it produces much more erotic and bearable sensations. Direct oral touch is fine for both the glans and the clitoris, however, but as we can't manage it for ourselves, I cover this in chapter 5.

Step 10: Be aware of how the steady pulsing action of your fingers is translating to every square centimetre over and around your clitoris. Keep your fingers moving around your vulva and Mount of Venus – the cushion of flesh over your pubic bone (see diagram on page viii) but always pause for longest just over the bud of your clitoris and its shaft on the slight ridge between it and your pelvic bone.

Step 11: Try using the pulsing and circling fingertip movement at a variety of speeds. Pressing or circling at intervals of about one second for a while, then increasing the tempo while keeping a steady rhythm but with no sense of hurry. You're not in a race – this is for the pleasure of the experience as a whole, not just reaching the finishing post.

Slow down for a while, then speed up again, seeing what effect it has on the sensations all around your vulva. Just go with the flow and find out what works best for you.

Step 12: Now and then stop the stimulation completely and just wait awhile, calm but alert. I find the sensation in my clitoris increases – sometimes almost immediately, sometimes after a minute or so.

Now tense the muscles, really squeezing the pubo-coccygeus muscle (often called the PC muscle) up, and rock yourself, with your thighs together, and your vulva and especially the shaft of your clitoris pressed against the heel of your thumb. Relax the muscles now and lie completely still for about 30 seconds.

Step 13: Rock some more and gently begin pulsing your fingertips again, concentrating now on your clitoris through its hood and the whole clitoral shaft. Use your wrist to press against your Mount of Venus, too, in the same action as the side of your hand. This is where your orgasm will gain strength. Focus on this area; feel it; let the energy of the orgasm build. Rock your pelvis up into your hand in a circular movement, mimicking your hand's. Press. Relax. Press. Relax. Arch yourself into the movement while you are doing this.

Step 14: Notice how the touch is now producing sensations not just where it currently is, but in other places too. Be very aware of the sensations in your clitoris, to each side of it (many women report the area just to the left of and slightly below as the most pleasurable places) and just above it, along the shaft.

Remember the clitoris is much, much larger than the bud itself – clitorally associated nerve endings extend way beyond it in all directions – and their boundary is probably still waiting to be fully discovered. See if you can register the arousal they're encouraging as the arteries bring blood and oxygen to the area, increasing the intensity of sensation and building sexual excitement.

Step 15: Throughout all this, you'll probably unconsciously contract the PC muscle that especially affects this whole area, but squeeze it consciously too as though you're stopping yourself from peeing. It feels like you're bringing your vagina up towards your clitoris and increases the stimulation to it and the whole vulva, particularly directly around the vaginal entrance.

Step 16: At the same time contract your thigh muscles, pushing your thighs together over your hand. Clench the muscles of your bottom, too, the ones in the cheeks and those around the anus. Squeezing yourself together like this in conjunction with the stimulation of your hand increases the sensations tenfold.

Step 17: Don't forget to breathe! This may sound silly but it's easy to get so carried away that you're snatching air in short, sharp breaths and this can mean you're not getting enough oxygen to help your orgasm – remember it's all aided and abetted by the increased flow of blood which carries oxygen to all the tissues. So keep breathing deeply, by all means, but make it regular. Remembering to do this, even at the height of the arousal curve, can actually make all the difference and help tip you over the edge into orgasm.

Step 18: You may find you orgasm almost immediately or very soon. But most likely it will take longer and be helped along if, after, say, 15 minutes of the exploratory and preliminary stimulation described above, you now change technique and begin using the heel of your hand. Place your hand on it's left edge (if you're using your right hand) between your legs along the length of your vulva with your wrist resting on your Mount of Venus so that the heel of your hand is lying against your clitoral shaft and hood, and your thumb against the rest of your vulva, just reaching the vaginal entrance. Now press with your hand, gently rocking it against you, so that again you're not rubbing but manipulating the skin and tissues of the clitoral hood and the inner and outer labia.

Step 19: Press, release, press, release and rock from side to side. Sometimes, instead of pressing with the side of your hand like this, press into your hand with your body.

Step 20: Squeeze those muscles, hug your hand and draw the pleasure upwards as though you're pulling it towards your stomach.

Step 21: When you can feel such intense sensations in and around your clitoris that it feels as though the crescendo has to peak, go for it, keeping the tempo steady and quite fast, arching your back with each press of your wrist, keening into the building climax. Don't hold your breath in excitement, remember to keep breathing – the oxygen will be circulated to the nerves and muscles and help enable orgasm.

When orgasm comes, let it. Just go with it – your body will react in its own way. Keep your body pressed against your wrist but stop all other action, poised in the pleasure.

If you don't come this time, don't go on for too long – enjoy the exercise for itself and after a maximum overall time of about 30 minutes, stop. Any pleasure fades in intensity after a while and so by containing it you'll come back to the exercise next time, looking forward to the fresh pleasure of a new session. This is also helpful in encouraging your mind and body to learn to go swiftly up the arousal curve and have an orgasm within the time frame.

Practise, practise, practise

You know, it's the strangest thing, but however much we want to learn, improve or just keep up a skill, and however much we enjoy it once we get going, we often don't make the time to practise and we even pass up spontaneous opportunities. Pleasuring yourself along the arousal curve and tipping over the peak into the most intense sensation of all may come naturally to some, but for most of us it's something to be learnt. It stands to reason that we're not going to get good at something unless we practise, but nevertheless we're often resentful when we don't practise and remain inept.

All I can say is if you're serious about being in control of your orgasms, you have to recognise that it's all down to repetition. It's about practising the basic method often – every day if you can manage it and at least twice a week – and enjoying it. If after a few weeks you haven't had an orgasm, it's up to you to read the rest of the book to discover and remove any causes that are deterring you and thwarting your quest.

If undertaken enthusiastically, this journey of self-discovery will revolutionise your sexiness and sensuality and you'll feel on top of the world both physically and emotionally. You don't have to have orgasms to feel delightfully feminine and sexually fulfilled and to thoroughly enjoy sex. As I've said before, orgasms are wonderful, but they're not necessarily intrinsic to great sex and vitality. Fantastic, pleasing, satisfying, certainly – but so is the whole arousal curve and your general feeling of well-being and happiness in your sexuality and sensuality.

Practise is key to orgasms – but do remember the pleasure it will give you is also valid and awesomely good just for itself.

How long will it take until I start having orgasms?

Like most abilities and skills, unless there are any factors affecting your orgasmability (we'll explore possibilities later in the book), your progress will depend largely on how often you practise and your individual natural sex drive and sensitivity at this time. For example, if you are a young woman who feels sexy and is very responsive to sexual pleasure but haven't quite got the knack of taking high arousal into orgasm, it might only take one or a few sessions to discover it and a few sessions more to grow your confidence and fluency. If you are going through a time of hormonal change, for instance, after having a baby, or have not given yourself sexual pleasure for some months or more, it could take many more practice sessions to coax your responses back to full-on vitality. On average, it will take around 12 to 15 practice sessions to develop your genetic sensuality and learn how to let it lead up the arousal curve and into orgasm.

What if I haven't had an orgasm by then?

Read any sections of the book that you haven't already, trying out the ideas and following my suggestions for removing any blocks stopping you from climaxing. As well as reading chapter 7, which covers health and well-being, I recommend seeing your doctor for a check-up to rule out any illness or condition that could be affecting your sexual responsiveness and, if you're currently on medication that may be having an effect, to discuss how this can be resolved. All being well physically, you may like to consider seeing a psychosexual counsellor.

Distraction therapy

If, after a few practice sessions of the basic technique, you're finding that you're not climaxing, or your orgasms have disappointed you, it may transform the situation if you pleasure yourself without focusing your mind on the sensations at all but on something entirely different.

Here are some suggestions:

- If you're doubtful that you'll be able to come, or would like a more powerful climax than you have experienced so far, let your hand pulse gently against your vulva while you read a book or watch TV – it must be something that fully engages your mind so that the feel of your hand doesn't subsume your concentration.
- Stop reading (or whatever it was you were doing) and completely focus on your hand's touch, and how relaxed and good you feel.
- Stroke yourself on your arms, the cheeks of your bottom, your temples, the sides of your neck – wherever you want – and feel each part of your body anticipate and respond to your touch.
- Move your hand into the basic technique again against your vulva, this time really focusing as you increase the

tempo and pressure and begin to move your pelvis in the rocking, circling motion against your hand.

- At the same time, bring a favourite fantasy to mind and let your mind and body lift you up the arousal curve as far as you want – having an orgasm if it happens or just enjoying the pleasure if you don't.
- Relax back into your book or other pastime, pleased with yourself and content.

This is marvellous for absorbing the fact that bodily pleasure is natural and non-threatening and very much a part of your capacity for pleasure generally. And because self-pleasuring while reading or watching TV builds arousal subconsciously, the shift into consciousness of the pleasure you're giving yourself has huge impact, often swinging you right up to the higher reaches of the arousal curve.

In summary: How to give yourself an orgasm

- Choose a comfortable, warm place where you won't be interrupted.
- Set the mood with low lighting, scented candles and music that makes you feel sensual and relaxed.
- Take off your clothes.
- Settle down in a position where you are well supported and can touch your vulva easily.
- Don't forget the lubricant!
- Throughout the rest of the steps, notice the different sensations depending on where you're touching and the kind of touch you're using. What's best? Which are your favourites?
- Now follow Step 4 on page 50 and onwards, reading as you go so you don't miss out any stage or suggestion. If you find it difficult to read and focus on your touch and sensations at the same time, read a step then put the book down while you practise it, then read the next one, etc. These pauses can be erotic in themselves as they tantalisingly delay gratification.

Chapter 4

Once You Get Going – Variations on a Theme

Like most new abilities, being orgasmic is best taken step-by-step. You learn a basic method, then you practise it. Then you learn another stage, and practise and so on, as your knowledge and skill increases and expands.

I remember learning to ski many years ago. Initially I found it extremely challenging, as it didn't come naturally to me at all. Whereas one or two people left our beginners' group within hours to join the improvers, it took me several sessions and much of the time I was thinking, 'I'll never be able to do this.' But by day six, perseverance saw me promoted to green run stage – a notch up from elementary but still pretty much for beginners. Not that I was displaying any flair yet but I was managing to safely get from the top of the slope to the bottom and having a lot of fun. On the last day of my trip green runs suddenly seemed ultra-easy. Next year, I promised myself, I would stay on green runs for the entire week, enjoying my new prowess. But two hours into the first day of that next trip they seemed much too easy and I was itching to go up a level. So another challenge, more lessons, more practice, and by the end of the week I'd progressed through blue to red runs and I was now an intermediate skier.

You'll experience similar learning steps and stages as you practise being orgasmic. All you want to do initially is have an orgasm. Then you want to prove to yourself you can do it again. And the next challenge after that will be to orgasm easily, whenever you want to. Once the basic method is thoroughly in your control, you look for variation, keen to try other ways, other speeds and to become more accomplished.

You may find that some steps or ways come easily to you, whereas others are more difficult. Remember that what seems impossible one day – so much so that you wonder if it's worth persevering – will probably, with practice, become easy for you within a few tries.

So, once you're good at orgasming when you're lying on your back, try self-pleasuring in a different position. Perhaps try lying on your side or sitting in a chair to start with. The general rule to stick to, as in the basic method, is if you don't climax within 30 minutes or so, think 'That was great anyway,' and call it a day – or, if you're very aroused, sink back into your now familiar beginner's position on your back and indulge yourself. The next few times you self-pleasure, practise in the new position. If, after a few times it's not doing it for you, that's okay – move on to something else and just use it occasionally for foreplay.

Even if you've no specific problems that lead you to consult other sections of this book, take a look anyway as there may be some scope to improve on various elements that affect your sexuality.

As you develop sexually, making love to yourself will seem more and more natural – just as another language suddenly becomes second nature, so does feeling personally sexy. In fact, being orgasmic is a kind of language – an interactive communication of nerves, hormones, muscles, your mind and your self-understanding. Practise and you'll get fluent. Develop the language and you'll improve the communication between all the different facets of being orgasmic and you'll enjoy it more and more.

Of course you may finally decide that the basic method is your absolute favourite and you're happy to focus on it forever. Lots of women do this but the broadness of the self-knowledge you've gained by exploring different avenues to orgasm will enrich your enjoyment of the simplest technique – and sometimes just thinking of one of the other ways you tried will add more excitement than actually doing it ever did.

The G spot and the V spot

We hear a lot about the G spot, and though personally I think it's a mite overrated, many women find stimulation there very erotic and orgasmic, so, by all means, try it. You'll find your G spot on the upper wall of your vagina approximately three to five centimetres from the entrance. It's easiest to reach it with your index finger. Massage it gently and see if you like the sensation. If you do, you may like to try using one of the little finger gloves, often called a clit stimulator (see Useful Resources on page 242), which gives your fingertip an undulating surface for extra effect. As ever, remember to use plenty of lubricant. You may find that stimulating your G spot manually yourself or with a dildo, or when your partner stimulates you there with his finger or naturally during intercourse (see chapter 5) adds an extra belt of power to an orgasm.

I'd just like to add that you shouldn't feel inadequate if you don't seem to have a sensitive area in the G spot region, or if it doesn't do much for you – some women are turned on by it, some not especially so, if at all, and some don't have a noticeably sensitive place in that area. It's good to remember that we're all different.

However, a much more useful place that I recommend paying attention to every time you self-pleasure is what I've named the V spot. This is where the Mount of Venus meets the pubic bone and the top of the clitoral shaft and is a much more arousing and accessible pleasure place that sex experts rarely mention (see the diagram on page viii).

To locate it, rest your hand on your lower abdomen so that the tips of your first and/or second finger are at the place where the outer lips of your vulva begin. You'll feel a slight hollow there as though made for this exact purpose — and who's to know, perhaps it was? Human bodies are so orgasmically beautifully made. I like to think that this little dip where a fingertip sits so comfortably — along with other similar areas around the body, like the one just below the voice box where our collarbone meets, and the little hollows just behind our ear lobes, for example — were given to us so we could enjoy finding and appreciating them now and then.

Not that you'll want to rest when you touch the V spot — just doing so can start waves of arousal down the clitoral pathway and on around the vulva. It's a very special place that invites you to press and release, press and release in the way of the basic self-pleasuring method you're practising in this section. Or you can even more gently awaken sexual expectation by simply stroking the whole Mount of Venus rhythmically in an upward action towards you or in a circular motion. However unpronounced, this movement pulls slightly on the skin and tissues of the V spot with a magically arousing effect on the whole of the clitoris.

But it isn't just at the beginning of arousal that the V spot is valuable – it gives a powerful surge of pleasure at any stage of the curve. With your wrist resting in the meeting place of the top of your leg and lower stomach, put your hand between your legs with the heel of your thumb pressing on the V spot. Now rock your hand and wrist from side to side or hold them still and press and/or rock your pelvis against them.

Scientists will say the V spot is part of the clitoris and it's certainly part of the whole network of arousal-inducing nerves in that area. I used to think that together with the Mount of Venus, it was just the area above the clitoris that announces the presence of our hidden pleasure zones, but then I realised that it's actually a huge source of pleasure both on its own and as a complement to them.

While the G spot comes into its own when you're having intercourse, the V spot is a brilliant source of arousal and orgasmic pleasure whether you're making love to yourself or with a partner.

Having multiple orgasms

I remember when I was at university, a male tutor told our class there's no such thing as multiple orgasms, and that if women think they are having more than one, they are simply mistaking waves of the same one for new ones. He would say I was encouraging a myth by telling you about them, and creating false expectations.

I beg to differ! I know from personal experience and the testimony of many women that it's perfectly possible for some women to have several individual orgasms. These can follow on, one after the other, with only very brief recovery periods in between of as little as a few seconds and up to a few minutes or so.

I think all women, even those just becoming orgasmic, are pragmatic enough to realise whether or not multiple orgasms are somewhere they want to go, and whether they are ready for them. Millie, a very orgasmic woman I was talking to one day, said that she climaxed easily and strongly but only once in any lovemaking session whether alone or with her partner. She said it was complete in itself and she wanted to enjoy letting the blissful feelings slowly ebb and had no inclination to repeat them immediately.

A lot of women will echo this. But there are also many of us who do have two or more orgasms, one after the other, and many others who, though happy with one, are intrigued by the idea of following up with another and maybe another and depending on how much time and energy you have, the number is really up to you.

How to orgasm again

Here's a simple method to see whether being multiply orgasmic is for you or not. If you're thinking, 'no – once is all I want', that's fine, just skip this next bit.

Step 1: When you've climaxed, keep your hand in the basic technique position and let it rest there for a few moments more.

Step 2: Keeping your body still, start to contract your PC muscle gently and be aware of the residual arousal – there's sure to be some.

Step 3: Now move the side of your hand – that is your thumb, the heel of your hand and your wrist – very gently, pulsing it gently against your vulva, clitoral hood and shaft and V spot. You may feel as though a new surge of pleasure is beginning.

Step 4: Pause all movement for several seconds to let anticipation build.

Step 5: Now, with your hand in the same place but keeping it still, begin rocking and circling your pelvis in a kind of belly-dance movement so that it presses rhythmically against your hand and wrist.

Step 6: Next, use your hand to vary the focus of the pressure at different places along the pleasure zones. What turns you on this time – is it your V spot, your clitoris itself, the clitoral shaft or the area around the entrance to your vagina? Or is the feeling centring inside your vagina? If so, it's probably your G spot that's the most aroused part of you just now.

Step 7: Stay with the focus that most responds. Push the area firmly against your hand and at the same time contract your PC muscle. Press, retreat, press, retreat – just rock yourself against your hand and, if it will, let the new orgasm come.

You may find that now, or over the next few months as you become increasingly easily orgasmic, that you hardly have to move at all for this second (or further) orgasm to sweep over you. The refractory time may be just enough seconds for the previous one to fade and for you to differentiate between them.

I guess this is advanced stuff – but sometimes we're ready for a new stage of a skill before we should be according to the textbooks. Go with the flow if you feel ready and it seems like a terrific idea. Why not?

Introducing other pleasure zones

So far you've concentrated on pleasuring your vulva and the clitoral area. Now that you're comfortable with that, introduce sensation further away and see which areas link up and intensify the genital pleasure.

You may find that your whole body becomes almost electric in response and, if so, you'll find that the slightest touch – stroking or pressing with your fingertips, or lightly running your nails over your skin – will heighten the arousal curve and perhaps trigger orgasm. Or, like most women, there may be just one or two specific areas which particularly turn you on. Breasts are usually thought to be the most sensitive and erotic part of a woman's body after the genital area but for most of us, though we may enjoy our breasts being stroked or fondled, it's the nipples that give the intense pleasure that can seem to have a direct line to the clitoris and/or vagina. Some women can actually have an orgasm purely through nipple stimulation and many more find that it greatly adds to genital pleasure, zooming them several notches up the arousal curve and, for some, triggering orgasm.

From my own experience and from talking with other women, I know that nipple pleasuring is powerful both as a prelude to arousal and genital stimulation and during arousal to enhance it, so I highly recommend that you regularly enjoy it. Start off gently and see what works for you – just go with the flow.

Complement arousal with fantasy

I'm loathe to suggest using fantasy very early on when you're familiarising yourself with the basic method of self-pleasuring. I'd sooner you focus solely on the physical sensations you're producing and follow intently your arousal curve, really living it. But there's no doubt that a fantasy you love can work wonders if you're stuck on the arousal plateau and seem unable to tip yourself over the edge into orgasm. So, by all means, use fantasy once you're past the first session where you need to focus on the sensations of the basic technique. Later, when you're confidently orgasmic, it's a great way to add variety and excitement. Most women say that their most intense orgasms involve an element of fantasising.

Anything that turns you on in the present, or has done in the past, can be used as a fantasy to escalate sexual pleasure. A fantasy that works for you can kickstart desire, arousal and/or climax. You can use it at any stage of the way. It could be a dream or a memory of an erotic sexual experience; it doesn't have to be lengthy – once you know the story or scene and the effect it has on you, just thinking of one or two of its most erotic moments may be all it takes to trigger a surge of feeling.

Fantasies can originate from a huge variety of sources. Personal experience, imagination, dreams, books, erotic magazines and porn. Trawl for things that do turn you on or once did and keep them in your mind's storehouse, ready to pull out whenever you want.

I had the same fantasy for years: Bella's story

For years, the fantasy that always did it for me was one that came to me when I was quite young. I don't know where it came from – possibly a film I'd seen, as it was as clear as scenes from a movie and was very vivid in my mind. As a teenager, well before I had any real sexual experiences, I'd day-dream the story for ages and it would arouse a kind of longing which, though unsatisfied in reality, I loved.

It wasn't until I was in my 20s that I started to masturbate, and then I soon found that if I used this story, I could recapture that amazing feeling of long-ing and, together with the new addition of real desire and arousal, go seamlessly into an orgasm. Until then, though I'd had some good sex with var-ious boyfriends, I'd never climaxed. I'll always be fond of that particular fantasy because it helped me discover how to have orgasms.

Find a fantasy that's a catalyst for your pleasure and have a good time practising allowing it to trigger arousal and orgasm. Most orgasmic women have a favourite fan-tasy or two up their sleeve.

Using an erotic dream
If you wake up still aroused from a sexy dream, don't let it fade – have sex there and then, whether on your own

or with a partner. Use the lingering sensations to carry you up the arousal path again. Add to this your self-pleasuring skill or your partner's lovemaking to bring you to a dreamy but very real climax.

Is a vibrator a good idea?

A vibrator is a great idea but I recommend first learning how to give yourself an orgasm by hand and, if you're in a relationship, letting your partner bring you to orgasm with his hand, mouth or body.

Why wait? Well, a vibrator, if it suits you (which it probably will), tends to bring you to climax very quickly because the sensations it produces are strong and dynamic. There's nothing wrong with that in itself, once you know what you're doing and are good at both pacing yourself and arousing yourself in different ways – then you'll be able to have orgasms with or without a vibrator as you desire. But before you've reached that stage, a vibrator could spoil you for more sensitive, finely tuned arousal curves and, as there's nothing as good as the climax that follows a long, slow, ultra-sensual curve, this would be a pity.

If you've practised the basic technique in chapter 3 for several sessions and haven't had an orgasm yet, then you may find using a vibrator heightens the sensations

and takes you into your first one. You may wish, understandably, to keep using one and this is fine – but I'd
like you to still practise using just your hand at least
occasionally to fine-tune your response.

Vibrators are useful, however orgasmically experienced
you may be, to speed up the arousal curve when you're in
a hurry or for any time when you can't be bothered to
fantasise and your orgasm is slow in coming. Some
women love them, while others prefer their own touch.

Using a vibrator: Trudie's story

I have three favourites that I occasionally use. They
all give me good orgasms, ranging from small tremors
to really deep, strong spasms of pleasure. It depends
on all kinds of things – my mood, the time of the
month, maybe even what I've been eating – just as
any kind of sex varies hugely from occasion to occasion. But I'm not inclined to use a vibrator every
time or very often – my own hand gives me the best
orgasms by a long margin.

Once you're easily orgasmic, it's really up to you whether
you use your hand or a vibrator.

Using a vibrator or dildo

The trick to using a vibrator or dildo most successfully is to think of it not as a penis substitute but as another hand whose gentle vibration can arouse all the nerve endings along the length of your erogenous genital area, from the Mount of Venus to the perineum. So don't use it like a penis inside you, but like the side of your hand against you. Hold it against your vulva and rock yourself against it. Follow the stop-pause-start suggestions as for self-pleasuring with touch. Sometimes lie still, focusing on the vibration or the feel of the dildo and your body's response. Sometimes press against it. Sometimes move your pelvis – just like you do with your hand.

And what if I want to use it for penetration?
Sure, if you can find one that you're comfortable with. Until you know what you like, it's best to start off with a smallish one with the texture of an aroused penis – quite firm but very slightly squidgy. The 'rabbit', which is popular with many women, might be a suitable choice as it has the advantage of offering dual stimulation – one promontory of it pleasures the clitoris at the same time as the other pleasures the vagina and the G spot. See Keeping your vagina stretchy on page 197.

What part does the G spot play when using a vibrator or dildo?

If you decide you do want to try to pleasure your G spot, a vibrator or dildo is the thing to use. The G spot is the sensitive area on the 'roof' of the vagina between three and five centimetres in. When stimulated, it can cause intense pleasure and trigger orgasm. The jury's out on whether it's an erogenous zone alone or part of the clitoral complex. Certainly it's well worth finding to aid your quest to being orgasmic. A curved vibrator or dildo is useful for this, as you can easily angle the curved end of it on to the upper wall of your vagina just beyond the entrance. You may be able to find and stimulate the G spot with your finger too, especially, as previously mentioned, if you've one of those latex finger stimulators whose undulating surface can be very effective (see Useful Resources on page 242). You may or may not like doing this or the feeling of it. If you don't, not to worry – it's not essential at all and many women have amazingly orgasmic non-penetrative solo sex.

Remember that for any sort of vaginal penetration it's essential to use generous lubrication and to keep it well topped-up. If you don't want the bother of re-applying purpose-made lubricant, just use some saliva but be aware that it dries out quickly so you'll need to do this quite often. Vaginal bruising and fissures caused by insufficiently lubricated penetration are painful and the latter can easily be infected so I can't stress enough that you should always use lots of lubricant.

Other sex toys

Sex toys can be great fun and add variety to arousal and orgasms. Many women have a vibrator or two to use on their own or with a partner and there are all kinds of other gizmos and gadgets available to add variety to your pleasure. It's very much a matter of personal choice and I recommend sending for a catalogue and browsing through it to see what, if anything, appeals to you.

Similarly, if you already like or would like to try looking at pornographic material, you may find it takes you quickly up the arousal curve as you view it or as you think of it at another time when you're having sex. As a general guideline, most women prefer soft porn. Do remember, though, that neither sex toys nor porn are necessary for fulfilling, fantastic sexual pleasure. Your own hand, or a partner's hands and body, are brilliantly designed to pleasure yourself and many extremely orgasmic women neither need nor want to use anything else – so don't feel you're boring if you choose not to.

Chapter 5

How to Have an Orgasm with a Partner

Once you can confidently give yourself an orgasm and know the kind of stimulation that most arouses you, you're all set to introduce the same enjoyment to sex with a partner.

As I said before in the self-pleasuring section, forget the feeling there's a pressing need to have an orgasm early on – there is no such necessity. You may have one or even several very early on in your lovemaking sessions or it may be many months of lovemaking before you do. Either way is equally good, as long as you enjoy the process.

One of my heroines, Shakti Gawain, once compared life to a huge, complex, beautiful painting. 'Life,' she said, 'is a work in progress.' Similarly, so is your sexual story. You will always be discovering more about your capacity for pleasure throughout the phases and stages of your life. As you mature and your self-knowledge develops, so will your pleasure and your orgasms. There will be peaks and troughs along the way, of course, but overall your wisdom about yourself will deepen, enriching your life and your relationships more and more as the years go by.

So take it easy. Don't feel you have to rush yourself. You are becoming orgasmic, so enjoy the journey. And when the time comes, as it will, take pleasure in being orgasmic.

Lubrication, lubrication, lubrication

I can't stress highly enough that for orgasmic sex your vulva needs to be well lubricated. It helps a lot when you're making love to yourself, but with a partner it's essential because they obviously can't tell exactly how their touch feels to you, so despite their best intentions, they may inadvertently cause soreness with their hand. And if there's any question of welcoming his penis inside your vagina, it has to be able to glide in or it will hurt and could easily cause damage.

If you're young or the menopause is still many years away, your body will probably create plenty of natural lubricant as you become aroused during foreplay. As ever, the more kissing and petting, the better. Even so, I recommend adding more before you guide his penis into you – you can't have too much. A simple way is to transfer some saliva with your hand to the entrance to your vagina and stroke it around and just inside. Then take some more and use it to generously moisten his penis, all around the glans and the whole shaft. Easier still, if you like giving him oral sex, moisten him directly with your mouth.

But if, like some women at any age and most peri- and post-menopausal women, you don't get very wet even when highly aroused, you'll need to keep some purpose-made lubricant such as KY Jelly or Ero (see Useful Resources on page 242) by you both before and during intercourse. Smooth on enough to make any touch – whether it's your partner's hands or penis – smooth enough to glide over the skin, causing only pleasurable sensation, no friction. Any time you begin to dry out, ask him to pause so you can put some more on – it only takes a moment if you keep the pot or tube of lubricant within reach.

Lube made me orgasmic: Kelly's story

I used to use saliva to boost my own wetness but it was never really long-lasting enough and I'd often get sore. I'd have been too embarrassed to use a lubricant and my first husband never suggested it. So I was surprised when John, my gorgeous fiancé, produced a tube of KY Jelly and put it on the bedside table before we started making love for the first time. He put some on me when he was about to start touching me down there – my clitoris and so on. He made it a part of his lovemaking so it didn't feel clinical in any way – it was rather erotic, in fact. Since then it's a regular part of our lovemaking. We always make sure his penis is nice and slippery before he goes inside me. During sex, if we're taking our time, I'll say, 'Hey, better put some more "gloop" on,' and he'll stop moving and pull out for me to do it – he says it turns him on that I'm so upfront about it. Neither of us is the slightest bit embarrassed as it's just a necessary part of our lovemaking. In retrospect, I see the dryness as being the main difficulty between my ex and me. I just don't get naturally wet like some women do, so intercourse was a problem for me. I was either sore or frightened of being sore so there was no way I could ever really enjoy it. The sensations now are just amazing because I can appreciate them to the full. They blow me away.

So decide before you make love next time to use lubricant. Whether you choose to do so discreetly or to make it an obvious and sexy part of your lovemaking is up to you. If he's never had a partner who's used lubricant and is naturally curious, tell him that if he loves making love, he'll love lubricant – it heightens the sensuousness amazingly. No good lover is going to have a problem with that.

Foreplay purely for pleasure

I love this account of what used to be called petting but now is boringly known as foreplay. As Marianne, a 50-something woman says, foreplay most certainly is anything but boring. And I tell you what, she's right – it's the key to fabulously orgasmic sex.

Foreplay is as good as sex: Marianne's story

I put the reason I'm so orgasmic down to the endless hours I spent petting when I was a teenager. Although it was the supposedly liberated 1960s, us girls were acutely conscious that we mustn't get pregnant (it was drummed into us by our anxious mothers) and at that stage it wasn't so easy to get the pill. The boys had also been indoctrinated that if they got a girl into trouble, they'd have to marry her. So we honestly – well most of us – didn't have sex. Instead we'd have amazing smoochy sessions of kissing – it was like an art form in itself – and explore each other's bodies. I would allow a boy to touch my breasts but that was about as overtly sexual as we got. When I was 16, my boyfriend, George, who was new to our crowd and more experienced than the other boys, added something to the usual pattern – he'd slip his hand between my legs when I was sitting on his lap and just press it against me. Some evenings a kind of electric pleasure would shoot through me in waves. I didn't know it was orgasm or even tell him about it, I just thought it was amazing. I never touched his penis – that would have been far too daring.

When I met the man who was to become my first husband, I sensed this would be my first serious relationship and that he'd be my first proper lover. Until he managed to get hold of the pill for me we just petted, but we went a lot further than I ever had before. We'd take all our clothes off whenever we got the chance and just adore the look and feel of each other's bodies. When he gave me an orgasm with his hand I finally realised what one was! As soon as I was on the pill, we made love properly. It was simple and straightforward but utterly amazing – we adored each other and we adored giving each other pleasure. I can't remember ever not coming with him. I always did, every time – until the sadness, years later, of making love for the last time when we were about to break up and were terribly upset. Silly young things – we should have stayed together. The wonderful lovemaking was such a great gift and we could have worked out the other differences that came between us.

I'm all for today's sexual permissiveness and decreased inhibitions. It's great that contraception is easily available and that the old double standard that it's okay for men to sleep around but not women has at least become less prevalent. But it concerns me that the carefree, prolonged petting described above has largely disappeared among single people of all ages when they're having casual one-off encounters. Among young people, particularly, one-night stands are acceptable, even expected. Yet the number of women who don't have orgasms is high. When having casual sex, we might get off on the excitement of it, but if it's too quick and not intimate, it doesn't help develop the kind of confident orgasmic self-knowledge that prolonged petting or foreplay nurtures. And when a casual one-off encounter develops into a steady relationship, the woman will expect and be expected by her partner to come as quickly as she did in their exciting early encounters. But many single people tell me that casual sex, though they feel it's the done thing, is orgasmically a non-event for them.

It's over too quickly: Lucy's story

It's too quick. Even if I'm mad for someone, I need a bit of time to get genitally aroused and I definitely need more than a few minutes of kissing, a bit of groping and then two or three minutes of inter- course. The men I meet don't want to hang about – they expect you to be up there with them and if you don't come by the time they do, tough.

If women go along with quick sex because they want to appear sassy and normal, it may explain why so many have never had an orgasm, or why often those that do soon find they no longer can once the excitement factor settles into the calm of a long-term relationship.

Of course not all newly together couples have quickie sex — many start off with slow, luxurious, sensual petting and continue to enjoy it, developing a fabulous sexual rapport that lasts throughout their life together. But with our lifestyles today and the common misconception that women 'get there' as quickly as men, all too often couples make love less and less and more and more perfunctorily. Even women who were initially orgasmic can then lose the knack, and those who never have been have little chance of discovering it.

We hardly ever make love: Susan's story

We only make love when we remember we haven't for a while and think we should. I know what he likes and he thinks he knows what I like, so it's quicker than it used to be. When he's about to come, he says, 'Are you ready?' and I say, 'Yes' and fake it because I'm tired and want to go to sleep. I haven't had an orgasm for months and the last few times I've managed to slow him down and tried, I haven't been able to. I think I've lost the ability. It worries me a lot.

The fact is, women need foreplay and we need lots of it. Sex therapists know this and use what they call 'sensate focus' to get couples used to touching and loving each other, and enjoying the immense range of pleasurable sensation this gives without any thought of direct genital contact or orgasm. If couples practise lots, like we always used to, and don't cheat by having intercourse or genital sex of any kind for ages until they really know each other and have established an accord, it works like a dream. The woman will gradually discover her capacity to receive pleasure with and from him, and when the time comes to go on to fully fledged genital touch, whether manual or oral sex or intercourse, chances are she'll be easily orgasmic.

The problem with sensate focus as a therapy is that couples tend to feel they're role-playing to please their counsellor rather than doing it for their own mutual pleasure. If you've missed out on petting in the past, or don't do it much or at all with your partner now, think of it as being an enjoyable interlude before you make contact sexually in any explicit way again. If you're in a relationship, make a commitment with your partner that for the next three months or so you're going to make the effort to pet every single day, and at the very least, most days. However busy you both are, find a slot and stick to it. Get to know every square centimetre of your bodies. Massage each other. Do those pressing, circling, stroking touch movements described in the technique sections, not genitally, but everywhere else on your bodies. Watch TV at the same time if you like — as long as you keep touching each other, whether taking turns or simultaneously.

Sensual massage: Kelly's story

Having my feet stroked, pressed and massaged is almost orgasmic for me. The pleasure is just blissful — I can't tell you how good it makes me feel. And yes, it does make me feel sexy, not in a 'must have' kind of way, but in making me feel as though my body is vividly alive — very aware and incredibly sensual. I feel very womanly, and very much loved by my man, which means I feel tender towards him too.

Postscript
Lucy decided that she would not have casual or quickie sex again with any new boyfriend.

No more quickie sex: Lucy's update

At first I had to summon all my assertiveness (not to mention my own willpower) to tell potential partners that I didn't have sex in casual relationships. I braced myself for them losing interest in me instantly or trying to persuade me to fuck but I was pleasantly surprised – only one dropped me and another said 'Come on, you don't mean it,' and tried to seduce me. Everyone else I had that initial chemistry with not only accepted what I said but seemed to be glad. I thought more of them, too – it created a very pleasant mutual respect I'd never experienced before. I had some fantastic snogging sessions and though some tried to put their hand between my legs and take things further, they were fine about it when I told them that wasn't the deal. Two of them didn't want to progress the relationship for other reasons, and I didn't want to with a third, but then we wouldn't have even if we had gone to bed together, would we? Then I met Stewart and we really clicked. I told him the petting-only rule, and he was fine with it. I've never been so relaxed with a man. After a while I had my first orgasm ever – I'd only ever faked it before. He was dead chuffed that he was my first! Now we have sex all the time but we always start off by petting. I never thought I could be so orgasmic but I am!

Susan also liked the idea of the petting programme. She told her husband about it and he wasn't surprised to hear that she'd been faking orgasms.

His side of events: Oliver's story

Actually I'm relieved to know that Susan had been faking orgasms. I thought sex had become mechanical for her and that her climax was a kind of reflex that more or less anyone could have given to her. I felt unimportant to her and it hurt more than I realised. Yes – it would be great to go back to the kind of sex we used to have. Susan is the most important person in the world to me – of course we'll make the time.

Pretty soon, Susan's once easy orgasms began to happen again through petting. Since then they only have intercourse if she's already come or is on the brink of it so that Oliver can hold back his own climax until she has hers. She's delighted they've a great sex life again and says a big plus is that she and Oliver have become romantically and sexually close again, as well as being 'a good working team'.

Ah, intimacy! A kind of mutual giving of tenderness and love as you pleasure each other in so many ways. It feels very, very good. And you have to be generous to each other, both in giving and receiving. Be generous and it will come back to you a hundred times more as you grow towards being orgasmic sexually as well as sensually.

Becoming orgasmic though his touch

When you're learning to be orgasmic with a partner through whichever medium – his mouth, his hands or his penis – you need to concentrate on the sensations he's giving you. So while he's pleasuring you, don't attempt to please him – lie back and enjoy what he's doing. Later you may find you can come as you return the compliment. During this probationary period try not to confuse your mind – take turns to give pleasure and, unless he's a man who is happy to make love to his partner after his own climax, agree that his turn at pleasuring you will be first.

To be honest, his touch on its own is probably the least likely way you'll orgasm as a beginner. But it's a very pleasurable, arousing part of petting and of course

I could be wrong – he may turn you on so incredibly that you are brought to climax straight away. If not, it's no problem at all because as long as he gets good at pleasuring you with his hand, even if you don't quite come, you'll be so aroused that he'll easily be able to tip you over the edge with his mouth or through intercourse, or alternatively you can masturbate for a few moments to launch yourself. So he needs to be an expert in manual technique and – as men rarely come to it naturally – the best person to teach him is you.

If you're still not sure what you like, re-read chapter 3. Then have a few sessions of self-pleasuring on your own, paying attention to what feels good, better, best and orgasmic. Note and memorise the exact amount of pressure you're using, repeating it on the back of your hand (not the palm as it's too sensitive) to help fix it in your mind so that you can show him what you like later by repeating it on his hand.

It's much easier to show your partner what kind of touch you like when you're familiar with your responses through your own touch. When you know exactly how to move your hand, you can show him precisely how it's done so he can do the same. He'll soon remember how to produce the same wonderful degree of arousal as you do for yourself, and in time, as you learn to relax with him and enjoy his new lovemaking to the full, you'll find you can let yourself go into orgasm just as easily as when you're alone. (If you find you have ongoing difficulty letting go enough of any persistent inhibitions or resistance to have an orgasm with him, psychosexual counselling will help and there is also a helpful book called *Women's Pleasure* by Rachel Swift with a useful section on this (see Useful Resources on page 242).

A key to helping him become a brilliant lover is to make sure he's fully familiar with your anatomy. The non-expert man is liable to think he's extremely experienced if he knows, or thinks he knows, where and what your clitoris is! If your man, like many, isn't absolutely sure what's where, show him. He needs to understand that there's more to the clitoris than the bud beneath its hood and you may need to enlighten him about the clitoral shaft and it's all-round extent. Show him the places that particularly turn you on to the side of the shaft and further down the vulva. And make it clear what an amazingly erogenous zone the Mount of Venus is and especially the V spot. As long as you're not patronising, he'll be delighted to have existing knowledge confirmed and extended – it feels great to be a good lover and the more knowledgeable he is, the better lover he'll be.

As you show him the way around this intimate area,

guide him to perfection with enthusiasm whenever his touch is pleasurable, and whenever he gets the pressure and/or movement the way you especially like it. Actually, even if you are lucky enough that he's a fantastic, experienced lover, you'll almost certainly have to adjust him slightly to your preferences, as each one of us is a unique being with different responses.

Don't tell him what *not* to do; rather, encourage him by expressing your pleasure when he gets it right. If you've had enough of something he knows you like, don't wait until it begins to annoy you – simply guide his hand onwards with yours. He'll soon learn how to vary how and where his fingers are moving, sometimes stroking, sometimes doing the pulsing, circling thing described in chapter 3. He may like to read that section himself and look at the diagram on page viii if he's not quite clear on what's where.

Another way to help him is to touch the tips of your first finger and thumb together and use the oval you create as a 'map' of your vulva. Show him exactly how you pleasure yourself in your favourite erogenous zones so that he can copy you. Better still, show him on *his* hand to demonstrate, and then let him try it out on your hand before he practises on your vulva. Actually, gently practising that gentle pulsing, pressing touch anywhere on your body is incredibly sexy and arousing as it creates anticipation of the real thing.

Dealing promptly with things you don't like

This is important as if you ignore it when he does something that doesn't please you or worse, hurts you, he'll assume you like it and keep it in his repertoire of touch. Gently but firmly stop the movement with your hand on his and indicate you want him to move on or guide him as to how you'd like him to vary what he's doing so that you do like it. If he continues to do something you dislike, tell him, but be sure to tell him as soon as you can when he starts to do something that you do like.

Touch through fabric

If you find his hand directly on your vulva too sudden or intrusive even when you're very aroused, try keeping your knickers on and let him caress you through them. Instead of desensitising you, you'll find the sensation this gives, though less intense, is deliciously exciting. What happens is that the cotton or silk has the effect of keeping the labia together and, as his hand moves, they move the whole area, gently pulling the clitoris and surrounding area and creating waves of subtle pleasure. You may like to try it yourself during your self-pleasure practice too.

General guidelines for your partner:

- No rubbing – it doesn't feel so good, plain and simple.
- No roughness of touch or pressure that's too firm, and absolutely no poking or scratching – think gentle, sensual but firm and positive.
- No inserting fingers into your vagina unless you like it. We can do it ourselves when self-pleasuring because we feel immediately if there's any soreness. A partner can't tell if their nail is a bit scratchy as it goes in. As I say, you may like it and, if so, fine. But unless you know you definitely do, I wouldn't take the risk of letting your partner try – it can be a real passion killer. Don't worry about missing out on the G spot. You'll orgasm very nicely without stimulating it and you'll have something to look forward to when you're having intercourse.

He touches me through my knickers: Sue's story

I don't know why but it turns me on far faster if I masturbate or he touches me through my knickers. It seems to have a great effect above my clitoris on my Mount of Venus, and when I feel myself beginning to get orgasmic, the feel of his hand (or mine) pressing through the material against the entrance to my vagina does the trick and I come very powerfully. Actually, this was how I had my first orgasm ever, so although I know how to come in other ways now, it's alway an extra-special technique for me that we often come back to.

Becoming orgasmic through oral sex

I only started having oral sex in my 40s: Nell's story

I read lots about oral sex when I was about 12 – it sounded inviting, to put it mildly. But somehow it wasn't until I was in my 40s, can you believe it, that I was confident enough to let a man go down on me. Even then, thank goodness my lover was extremely experienced and knew how good it would feel for me, otherwise I'd probably have gone on forever pretending it wasn't my thing when I hadn't even tried it. He told me his ex used to like it better than anything else, and as he was an amazing lover generally, I have to admit I was very curious – but self-conscious and embarrassed nevertheless. So without further ado he dived under the bedclothes and did this very, very gentle thing to me. It was astonishing – like nothing I'd ever felt in my whole life. It was like being kissed with a soft flow of warm water, like waves lapping on a shore. So soft and silky I can't tell you. It was a kind of heaven and then the waves of orgasm began and I had one of the deepest, longest ones ever.

Many women in their 50s tell me a similar story to Nell's. Younger generations are thankfully far less inhibited, but even so many women of all ages have told me they've discouraged their partners as they thought they wouldn't like going down on them. If you have held your partner back from cunnilingus, do let him show you what it's like.

How to Have an Orgasm with a Partner

Let's be honest: oral sex is fantastic for women when it's done well and yes, most of us would like it to be part of lovemaking. If your partner's happy to oblige (and most men are when they find out it's easy – actually a lot easier than manual stimulation – and not scary at all), put any negative feelings you have about it on hold, give him the go-ahead and lie back and enjoy. First, though, to allay the common fear that we'll be smelly, it's more important than ever to wash just before we make love, just as you'd expect him to, especially if you're going to give him oral sex. Sure, the scent of sweat can be very sexy and a turn on, but only if it's fresh, untrapped sweat and you really like each other's natural bodily scents.

The only thing you need to remember about receiving oral sex is to keep in a position that's comfortable for him and to resist the probable urge, when you're on the verge of orgasm or during it, to bring your legs together.

Lie on your back and draw your feet up towards you and widen your knees apart as far as they'll comfortably go – this way he can kiss and caress you with his mouth without feeling claustrophobic. It will be easiest for him if he kneels or lies between your legs, facing you. He may find it easier still if you slip a pillow under your bum to lift yourself a few centimetres towards him.

Then enjoy the sensations he gives you. If you're tense — as is absolutely natural if you're not used to oral sex or have been embarrassed by it in the past — tell yourself, just as you would if you were having a foot massage for the first time, that you are going to relax and enjoy it. Remember that he wouldn't be doing it if he didn't want to and if he happens not to like it, he needn't ever do it again, so don't spoil everything by worrying about him. Now focus and let yourself go with the flow of the pleasure.

If you find you're feeling orgasmic but aren't quite getting there, stroke or gently squeeze your nipples and, without moving your hips (stillness is important as it will be uncomfortable for him otherwise) contract your PC muscle. At the same time, bring your favourite fantasy to mind.

Fantasy's the key: Rachel's story

I can be lying there thinking, 'This is very nice but it's not turning me on – I'm not going to come like this.' And then I'll start playing with my nipples, or rather, my right nipple, which for some reason is more erogenous than the other one. Suddenly I'm much more responsive down below – it's as though there's a direct line to my vagina and clitoris. Sometimes that's enough to make me orgasmic, other times I add a fantasy. Again, it's like a boost of erotic energy and usually all it takes to make me climax for real.

If you don't climax within a few minutes, that's fine – lots of women don't during oral sex, and many others would take too long for comfort for the man. Giving oral sex, as you probably know well from doing it for your partner, is about the most unselfish thing you can do in bed as the person receiving it is passive and needs to focus dedicatedly.

Final note
If oral sex just isn't your thing, no matter how good at it he gets, tell him the truth. He won't mind in the slightest not having to do it any more. But do give it a fair trial – most of us, once we relax and let go to the pleasure, adore it.

Tips for your partner

- Aim for the moist, licking, lapping effect described at the beginning of this chapter. Usually, when kissing mouth to mouth, saliva would be a turn-off but in cunnilingus it's great in helping that warm and soft feel you want to achieve.

- It's a myth of oral sex that your tongue needs to go inside her vagina — it doesn't at all. Of course you may like to try it and if she likes it a lot, that's fine. But what most women love best is the lapping, licking effect that, though subtle, often produces extraordinarily deep waves of pleasure.

- Keep your tongue soft and be very careful to keep your teeth out of the equation. (You may think this is obvious, but it's surprising how many men think women like to be nibbled. We don't.)

- She may prefer you to stay with a general caressing of the whole vulva from vagina to V spot, including the inner and outer labia, clitoris and clitoral shaft. Or, if she likes it, you can rhythmically and quickly lick her clitoris using an up and down or sideways movement, either directly or through the hood as she prefers.

- You can use your hands to gently press the labia together over her vulva and run your tongue gently along the groove or 'join' in the middle. Like stroking through knickers, the subtlety of the feeling this produces can take her straight up the arousal curve to the orgasmic plateau and very quickly thereafter into climax.

- She may not come so if she doesn't start becoming orgasmic after a few minutes, give her a last, lingering caress and then move back to a side-by-side position. This may be a good time to stop lovemaking while you feel very close and loving and orgasms can wait until another day. If she's extremely aroused, you may want to continue petting or maybe she'll ask you to go inside her — play it by ear.

Becoming orgasmic through intercourse

Let's get straight to the most sure-fire way to have an orgasm during intercourse. It's a variation on a traditional theme but with a particular movement that makes a tremendous difference to its orgasmability.

The way you're most likely to start having orgasms during intercourse is in what's known as the missionary position – you lying on your back with your partner on top, facing you; your legs wide apart with your knees drawn up towards you; him lying or kneeling in between them. Get the missionary position right – and all it takes is a bit of subtle adjustment to the way your bodies lie and move together – and all else being well, you'll have orgasms while he's inside you.

I'm going to start right from the beginning as even highly sexually experienced people can have gaps in their knowledge which make intercourse less fabulous than it should be. If you and your partner know most of it, please skim through the next two sections anyway, just to make sure there's nothing to learn.

He takes the weight – not you

You wouldn't believe how many women have told me they don't like the man-on-top position because their partner's too heavy. Excuse me? How can a man possibly not realise that being squashed underneath hundreds of pounds of body weight is not conducive to their partner's enjoyment? But there you go – some men either haven't thought of this, or don't care. If he puts his weight on you, do whatever it takes to get him off. All he has to do is to remember to support himself on his forearms. Some men find it more comfortable to kneel, or half kneel, to distribute their weight, rather than keeping their legs straight so their arms take most of their weight. Opponents of the missionary position say this is a disadvantage because the man can't caress his partner with his hands. But it's a great position to kiss and, anyway, when you're doing it well you will be in such a state of ecstasy that you won't need manual or any other stimulation.

Getting inside

Don't even think of letting him go inside you until you're well and truly aroused. Being wet isn't enough; the vagina, though extremely stretchable, often produces its own lubricant well before it relaxes enough to accommodate a penis. When you can easily slip your first and second finger in, you're ready – not before. As I discussed in detail in the section on lubrication (see page 85), if you're not dripping wet with your own slippery fluid, you'll already have applied some KY Jelly or similar lubricant liberally to the whole of your vulva before you started making love. Apply some more now, or if you're naturally wet, add some saliva just to be sure you're seriously slippery. Take special care of the entrance to the vagina and the perineum as it's easy to get painful fissures here too if the skin isn't moist enough.

Now take his penis in your hand and guide the head of it to the entrance of your vagina. Never, ever, let him push on in of his own accord. While not wanting to hurt you, his penis can't tell if it's catching on the skin connecting the entrance to the perineum and one push too hard or fast or insensitively can tear this delicate skin. If it tears, it will take days, possibly weeks, to fully repair and regain its suppleness and it won't do anything for your eagerness to have intercourse again. So guide him in slowly. It makes sense. If you're tensing your PC muscle, breathe in and then out, consciously relaxing it. Your mantra is: 'Let go. Relax.'

Another plus of holding his penis as you guide it in is that you can control the speed at which he enters once he's past the opening. A quick thrust to barge in isn't, contrary to popular male opinion, what you want even now. It could still stretch the entrance too much too soon, or he could knock against your cervix. So continue to introduce him positively but slowly and cautiously, enjoying the sensation of him inside you as he goes in, and gradually sliding your hand back to give him access. The minute you feel him touching your cervix or the end of your vagina, keep your hand where it is on his penis to stop him going any further. Keep it there until he's got the idea of how far he can go and you feel you can trust him not to push in too far for comfort.

My husband's too big for me: Billie's story

My husband's penis isn't particularly long – he's about 12 centimetres erect – but the problem was more its girth – it's much wider than any of my previous boyfriends'. There's no way he can get inside of his own accord as I haven't had kids so I'm quite tight. But it's absolutely fine because he lets me guide him in. He says it's like manoeuvring a car into a narrow space – a matter of patience and skill. He always makes me laugh, saying, 'Gently does it… slow but sure… ', and then he gives a big gasp of pleasure and satisfaction when he's safely in. He does fit right inside me but even so I tend to keep my hand nearby so that if he's getting too enthusiastic about thrusting, I can slip it around him and hold him back a little. He says that's sexy and doesn't have a problem with it.

(Once Billie learned about CAT, she rarely had to
hold him back like this once he was safely in – but
we'll get to that in a minute...)

A relatively slow speed of his movement in and out is
crucial to your pleasure. On the point of orgasm, some
women like the man to thrust rapidly whereas others
find it's a sensual all-but-stillness that does it for them
best – just do whatever feels best.

Okay – now you're ready for the crucial adjustment.

The key to a woman's climax is CAT

CAT stands for 'clitoral alignment technique'. My first
husband and I first read about it in an article in *Cosmopolitan* 30 or so years ago and exclaimed, 'That's what
we do!' I've never heard the term since but I can tell you,
as we'd discovered by chance, it's the best ever refinement to the good old missionary position.

How CAT works

Your partner, once his penis is inside your vagina, keeps
it there but moves himself forwards towards you a little
so that his pelvis – the part of his lower stomach area a
few centimetres up from the beginning of his penis – is
directly over and in contact with your lower pelvis and

Mount of Venus. Yes, it will mean he has to withdraw his penis a little, but he'll find he can comfortably keep much of it within you. Then he moves back to go deeper into you again, and then out a little to return to the pelvic touch, and so on – repeating this pattern just as he would normally go in and out during intercourse but with this slight forwards and backwards movement going on at the same time. Moving this way means that you are stimulated from your vagina all along your vulva to your clitoris and forward, even further, along the clitoral shaft to the Mount of Venus; as this is his main resting place before he moves backwards again, it ensures the V spot gets a lot of subtle attention causing, along with all the other sensations along the way, the most amazing mix of pleasure. It's easy, extremely comfortable, and I think the most arousing position of all.

This is an excellent position for moving in harmony. As long as he's taking his weight on his forearms, you'll be able to move your pelvis up and down and from side to side, maximising the wealth of sensations. Think of the circular, classic belly dancer rolling movement if you like, or imagine the kind of movement that keeps a hula hoop spinning round you. It won't be an effort at all because it adds hugely to the pleasure. He'll love it too – men consider pelvic movement very sexy.

I asked a friend what he specifically meant when he mentioned a new girlfriend was 'good in bed'. At first he looked puzzled and finally he said: 'It isn't that she's athletic and performing amazing gyrations or anything – we've actually had quite quiet, straightforward sex so far. But even in the classic position with me on top, she moves incredibly sexily. My last girlfriend used to lie completely still so it always felt it was completely up to me to please her as well as myself. She said she enjoyed sex but you wouldn't have known. There's no mistaking Carly's pleasure – she moves really sensuously in time with me – it's like a very exciting, amazingly erotic dance.'

Enjoy this movement for up to ten minutes or so. He can increase or decrease his speed but occasionally it's essential that he slows right down for the movement in both directions, so that you can fully take in the different sensations that each stage of the way produces.

Have him stop occasionally too, sometimes when he's deep within you, when you can lift yourself up to him and take him as far inside you as is comfortable and squeeze him with your PC muscle. And at other times, when your pelvises are touching, you can arch your pelvis up to meet him and press against him which will add extra-pleasure to your Mount of Venus, V spot and the clitoral area generally.

A big plus of this technique, besides being arousing and probably orgasmic, is that neither of you have to 'perform' – your bodies are moving in unison to produce a symphony of pleasurable sensations for you both and, quite honestly, you don't need anything else.

However, if he's athletic enough to kiss and gently suck your nipples, and for you to kiss on the mouth if you'd both like to (some people find this distracts their minds too much from the concentration needed to flow with the arousal curve), then that's fine. And, of course, once he's got the idea that he mustn't go further inside you than is comfortable for you, your hands are free to pleasure him in all kinds of ways if you feel like it. If it doesn't distract you too much either, lots of men love the cheeks of their bottoms being caressed, for example, or to have their partner hold him there and steer him through the movement.

If you are stuck on the arousal curve or orgasm plateau...

Remember, if you want to up the arousal level because it's not increasing or perhaps it was but now you're stuck on the orgasm plateau, stopping, waiting and feeling, then resuming movement may take you over the edge.

Moving beyond the arousal curve:
Meya's story

If I'm enjoying myself but not becoming orgasmic, I love Tony to suddenly hold still – either when he's deepest inside me or when he's edged up and is pressing against my clitoris and V spot. I'll lift my pelvis up towards him and circle a bit – like a belly dancer. It feels fantastic. Holding myself against him like this takes me straight to that last stage just before orgasm and sometimes I'll come right then. Other times we'll start moving together again and almost immediately I'll say, 'Yes, I'm ready now' and he'll move into me faster and let himself come with me.

This is the best position and way to orgasm simultaneously. A variation on this theme is to ask him to pull out of your vagina, pause for a while, and then guide him back in and move very, very slowly or, again, hold still for a few seconds more.

An instant orgasmic turn-on for most of us is to bring a favourite fantasy to mind. It also helps greatly to breathe deeply. It's surprising how many people forget to breathe at all for a few moments when they're approaching orgasm, but holding your breath actually impedes orgasm, which needs oxygen to work well. This is why knowing lovers tend to breathe heavily or even gasp air into their lungs as they're nearing climax. A few deep breaths can make all the difference, releasing extra oxygen into your bloodstream en route to the erogenous zones and especially, of course, to the clitoral area.

If he finds keeping his leg weight on his knees uncomfortable, it will help to put a pillow under your bum to lift your pelvis up towards him.

Great sex muscle control

'Uh, huh', I can hear you saying, 'you mean pelvic floor exercises, don't you? They're boring and such hard work – why bother!'

Well the good thing about pelvic floor exercises (often referred to as Kegel exercises) is that you can do other things while you're practising. Hard work? Actually you'll find they're really easy and it's just a case of remembering to practise for a few minutes each day. Why bother? Because taking control of your muscles down there will help you have stronger orgasms with or without a partner, maintain control when you have them and will also determine whether or not you can go multiple.

So let's get going. There are three areas of muscles to concentrate on:

- The PC muscle that affects the vagina and the perineum.
- The anal sphincter muscles around the back passage.
- The urinary tract muscles.

While you're reading this, try contracting them. The best way to do this is to imagine you're squeezing the walls of your vagina together, then that you're stopping yourself from passing a motion, then stopping yourself from weeing.

It may feel as though the contraction is all the same as when you tense one set, you tense all three, or you may find you can, straight away or with practice, feel each muscle group contracting – either way is fine.

Now repeat this exercise again and again, and in between tensing them, relax them. That's enough for the first few times. Once you get the hang of it, aim to repeat the exercise about three times a day for a few minutes at a time.

A good tip another sex counsellor told me is to think of it like going up in a lift. Clench your muscles as though you're lifting them up to the first floor and pause, holding them there. Then lift again, taking them up to the second floor. Pause. Then up again, as high as you can, to the top. Then let them all go and relax.

The first important point to remember, to encourage good muscle tone, is to go right through the stages of 'lift'. Put some energy into it and make sure you go to that last stage when you really clench the muscles as much as you can. The second thing to remember is to do the exercise frequently. Whenever you're sitting en route somewhere in a car, bus, train or plane, you can do it. No one will know. Or when you're at work or doing the housework, or listening to music or in the theatre – whatever. It only takes a few minutes and by doing it several times a day your muscles will become toned and ready to help you enjoy sex and orgasms to the full.

I can easily climax: Ellie's story

I used to do pelvic floor exercises because I read that it would be good for my partner during intercourse. I prided myself on being able to squeeze him with my vaginal muscles when he was inside me. He loved it. But then I found that by tensing the muscles, I could increase my own pleasure, whatever he was doing, and while I masturbated too. I've now found that if I'm really aroused and have that 'I want to come but can't quite get there' feeling, tensing the muscles a few times can bring me to climax. Now I know what a help they are, I'm going to make sure I keep the muscles in good shape for the rest of my life.

It's a good idea, it's easy, free – and it's helpful. What's not to like?

The G spot

As far as self-pleasuring is concerned, and manual and oral sex with a partner, the V spot is far more significant for orgasm than the G spot. But the G spot does come into its own during intercourse. The missionary position combined with the CAT technique is perfect for pleasuring it because the amount of penetration during much of the movement is probably only five to eight centimetres maximum, so the head of the penis will press against it perfectly, much of the time.

As mentioned in chapter 1 there's an ongoing debate about whether vaginal and clitoral orgasm are really disparate entities. Most women who regularly make love with their partner this way will soon learn they are. The sensations of a clitoral orgasm are – well – clitorally located, and a vaginal orgasm clearly comes from within the vagina. Close, certainly, and should they combine to make you come at the same time, impossible to differentiate because you'll be totally overwhelmed. But they are definitely two distinct types of orgasm.

Once you're used to having orgasms easily, when you're on your own, try having four in immediate or daily succession, triggering each with the pressure of your touch in a different place – focusing it on the G spot, clitoral shaft, directly over the clitoral hood or the entrance to your vagina. Notice where you have the crescendo of feeling as you climax. Interestingly, you may find it's not in the same location as the stimulation.

While the types of orgasm may be clearly differentiated, don't worry if they're not – for many women the sensations of orgasm seem to emanate from the whole of the vulval area from the V spot to the perineum and including the vagina. They are all associated with the clitoral nerve network which is much further reaching than the clitoris and clitoral shaft itself, and refer, or connect, to the nerves in all the erogenous zones.

Timing

I've mentioned climaxing simultaneously and yes, when it happens to you and your partner you'll feel fantastically intimate and very in accord. But, hey, it's only a matter of timing and once you're both familiar with each other's orgasmic paths, you'll soon be able to do it easily. Don't feel you always have to try to come together – it's nice when it happens spontaneously or if you particularly want to, that's all.

It depends on your partner: Tricia's story

When I was first with Bob, I'd never had an orgasm and it was a while before I started to. He was happy to give me as much time as I wanted and never tried to rush me. Then, when I grew confident at climaxing, he'd still always wait for me to reach that final stage and then he'd let himself go and come with me or soon afterwards. So I never had to gauge when I was going to come – I'd just enjoy myself and let it happen naturally. Now I'm with Stephen, it's very different. He's not as in control of himself as Bob was and he'll suddenly get to the point of no return and just climax with no warning. Fed up with being left up in the air because, once he's come, he just wants to sleep, I realised I'd have to look after my own path to orgasm myself. So I'd ask him to keep going with whatever we were doing – I particularly like it when he puts his whole hand sideways between my legs as he has this knack of swivelling the base of his hand against my clitoris and public bone, which is just magic, until I could feel myself getting near climax. Only then would I let him enter me with his penis and, when he had, he knew to keep almost still so that he didn't become orgasmic too soon and I could just move myself around and against him until I did. So sex is quite different from how it was with Bob, but just as brilliant in its own way.

You and your partner will have your own unique way of relating to each other as sexual partners. He might be the choreographer, or it might be you. Or perhaps you simply dance together in accord, with no need for direction. And you may find that coming simultaneously isn't as desirable for you as having your orgasms individually, in which case your preferred pattern may be for you to come first, then him, or the other way around (for lots of men, unlike Tricia's second partner, as mentioned above, are happy to continue making love to their partner after their climax).

We climax without each other: Mandy's story

We do sometimes climax together, but, quite honestly, although we feel very close, it's rather a surface kind of orgasm when this happens, perhaps because it's difficult to concentrate entirely on mine when I'm so aware of his. What I like best is when I come first. The waves of it are deeper and more intense and seem to go on and on instead of being just one sensation.

Another nice thing about coming first is that you can have more orgasms as he's en route to his own climax – and another one with his if you like. If you're reading this thinking, 'Damn, I haven't even had one orgasm with a partner yet,' don't feel daunted – be inspired. Once you've had one, you'll have learnt how to do it and from then on you'll practise the 'bringing yourself to orgasm' technique and the 'having an orgasm with him' technique until you're so fluent at the language of orgasmic sex that the art of timing will be second nature.

The missionary position with CAT is as good a position for practising timing as it is for practising the basic skill of having easy orgasms.

Other good positions

Once you are confidently orgasmic in the classic missionary position in conjunction with CAT or if for some reason it's not doing it for you, you can test-drive as many positions as you like. The Kama Sutra is fascinatingly comprehensive or you can consult any good book on sexual technique, or simply have fun using your imagination.

Sitting on the edge of the bed

Your partner should sit on the side of the bed facing inwards – his bum on the edge, his legs stretched out straight in front of him towards the centre of the bed. You sit facing him astride his lap with your legs dangling over the edge of the bed. Unless the bed is low enough for you to be able to put your feet on the floor, you won't be able to move your hips back and forth of your own volition but you can rock together in tandem.

Sitting on a chair

Similar, but more preferable for you because it produces the most amazing sensations, plus it's less of a strain on his back.

Get him to sit on an armless chair that's narrow enough for you to sit astride him, face-to-face.

Both this position and sitting on the edge of the bed are fantastic positions for you to orgasm. However, they're not so hot for your partner because he won't be able to move much and will probably become uncomfortable quite quickly, especially with the first one on the bed as there's nothing to support his back. Nevertheless, he will probably be happy to do these positions now and then because not only will it drive you wild, you'll orgasm in double quick time so he won't need to bear it for long anyway.

Why are they so good for a woman? Because he is inside you just a comfortable amount and possibly not too erect after the initial excitement, as this is a passive position for him, so you'll feel him pressing against your G spot. At the same time the whole of your vulva is naturally resting on and pressing against his lower abdomen because of the weight of your legs. As well as this you can kiss and hug and he can kiss your nipples too. All you have to do is squeeze your PC muscle and you'll have the most exquisite sensations ever.

Lying facing each other on your side
Put your up-side leg over his hip, and manoeuvre as necessary to slip his penis inside you. This is really good because you are then both free to move gently and sensuously, again with his pelvis pressing against your Mount

of Venus and V spot and spontaneously subtly stimulating the whole clitoral area. As in the above positions, he
may not come like this. Though this is not as stimulating
for him as it is for you, he'll probably be happy to stay
like this for some time while you slowly but surely go up
the arousal curve and into orgasm.

The starfish

You lie on your back with your partner to your right. He
should be on his side, facing you. You lift up your right
leg so that he can slot his right leg underneath it and
over your left leg, positioning him so that he can slip his
penis into you (you won't be able to guide him into
you). As far as your concentration is concerned, you'll be
very passive and able to focus purely on the sensations of
his penis inside you and his thigh perhaps pressing
against your vulva. Another plus point is that your hands
are free to self-pleasure your clitoral area as you wish.
The downside to this position is that it can feel a bit too
detached unless you're very confidently intimate with
each other already.

What about other positions?

Until you are having orgasms easily, I suggest just practising with the positions I have outlined above as, in my

experience, they are the ones that will bring you to climax most easily. This is not to say that you will not orgasm in the woman on top, rear penetration, anal sex or other positions – many women can, and do. But for now, while you're becoming orgasmic, they probably won't be very effective. The positions listed above are the most certainly orgasmic ones, the winner being the missionary using CAT – the clitoral alignment technique (see page 114).

Should you use fantasies and play them out with your partner?

This is a very, very personal and sensitive issue. Yes, I definitely recommend using fantasies once you're past the initial practice sessions in chapter 3. They're very erotic and a useful trigger for desire, arousal and climax. Whether to share them with your partner and perhaps play them out together is a very individual question. Some couples love to and if it turns you on or adds to existing pleasure at any stage of the arousal curve and doesn't upset either of you, then, by all means, act your fantasy out. But if you or your partner isn't happy with it, it could be a big turn-off for them, so obviously it isn't a good idea and, in that case, the person keen to use a fantasy is best to just imagine it.

Fantasy helped me to orgasm: Aakarshan's story

After trying and failing to have orgasms for several years, I discovered how powerful fantasy can be. I'd been with the same partner for months and sex had got a bit boring – to be honest I'd come to the conclusion I was never going to come and had switched off. But I wasn't ready to give up on the relationship as it had so much going for it. So one day I was pretending to be enthusiastic while making love and I started thinking about the book I was reading, which had some very explicit sex scenes. It was as though something switched on in my genitals and I was shot through with pleasure, which built and built until it exploded in ecstasy. After that, I soon learnt to harness the feeling without necessarily using that fantasy or another one. But I love using a fantasy sometimes because it allows me to experience a range of experiences that I wouldn't want to have in real life. Casual sex, for instance, just isn't me – I love my partner and I'm totally faithful to her – but I can imagine going with other women and men without her knowing and without hurting her. I usually only use a fantasy for a few moments to speed up getting turned on if I'm a bit slow, or to tip me into an orgasm if I'm hanging on the brink. If I want to run through a complete fantasy, I do it on my own as I'd feel disconnected from her if I used it while making love with her and that wouldn't be fair.

Sex got boring: Dae's story

For years I didn't need any stimulation other than my husband. But life became more complicated and we became more like friends and business partners than lovers. I stopped having orgasms and often couldn't be bothered to make love at all. But I loved him and we didn't want to break up so we went for counselling. I ordered one of the books you mentioned on fantasy and, unbeknown to my husband, settled down one free afternoon to read it. At first I thought it was a load of rubbish, but then I realised that I was getting physically aroused nevertheless, so I read on. In fact, there was only one fantasy in that entire book that had a strong effect on me – but goodness it was very strong. It was as though I'd been in the story – as though I was the central character but at the same time being turned on by watching her. Very strange but incredibly exciting. I had to stop reading to concentrate on self-pleasuring and almost immediately felt that intensity of feeling I hadn't had for months building. I stopped, waited, then started again and let go and it was like a wave of pleasure pressing on my clit and imploding.

It brought back my sex drive and my husband luckily didn't need any encouraging – he'd been missing sex a lot, it turned out, but hadn't liked to pressure me. I've 'collected' a couple more fantasies that work well since then, but that first one will always be special.

Enough advice on becoming and being orgasmic for now. You have a lot to practise and enjoy – probably enough for at least a year or so, and actually enough to have a wonderful love life forever. Of course once you're having orgasms confidently, you can go on adding to your sexual knowledge, mutual understanding and skill as much and for as long as you wish to.

Chapter 6

Making a Relationship a Great Place for Orgasms

We women expect a lot from our relationships, orgasm-wise. Whether or not we've had orgasms on our own, we hope or assume we will when we're in a relationship. And if we are confidently orgasmic in a relationship, it doesn't occur to us that we may not always be.

So when you find yourself still unable to have an orgasm even though you're now with someone, or when the tried and tested orgasmic lovemaking with your partner suddenly fails to take you into climax, it's both disappointing and worrying.

Why can't you have orgasms when you're with a perfectly nice partner who knows what he's doing and is a capable enough lover? It's a huge question with myriad potential answers. If relationship issues are causing your orgasm block, while just one issue may be apt for you, quite likely several will apply and need to be resolved. But first, it's essential to realise that it may not be anything in the way you interact generally that's causing orgasms to be absent. Only once you're confidently orgasmic on your own and have practised the most orgasmic techniques with your partner but still find you're not having orgasms should you start considering the possibility that interaction difficulties with your partner are blocking your ability to have orgasms.

Creating the right circumstances – just like on holiday

Because you want to get good at having orgasms when you make love with your partner, you need to practise often – and to practise, you need to make love. I'd recommend at least once a week, preferably twice. But often, once a couple are over the honeymoon phase of their relationship, they'll find themselves making love less and less.

My best advice to couples who like making love but rarely do so, or whose lovemaking tends to be a quick fix rather than the sensuous, loving experience that will help you become orgasmic, is to create the same conditions for mutually enthusiastic sex that you experience on holiday.

People sometimes ask me why it is they have fabulous sex with their partner when they're on holiday that's much, much better than sex at home. And why they orgasm so easily when they're away, too.

The reason is simple enough: on holiday you're relaxed and you're getting on well. You want to — and do — make love leisurely (because of the ample time), passionately (because being warm and sun-drenched makes you feel sexy) and very pleasurably (because time and passion complement each other to make you aroused).

Wouldn't it be nice if you could have such brilliant orgasmic sex at home, too? Well you can with just a little thought to create the right ambient conditions if you keep the holiday analogy in mind. Although you can't create exactly the same circumstances you can pick up on the key factors that make sex so easy and orgasmic as on holiday. Putting these into practice as a real ongoing part of your life is simple — you just need to decide to go with them. There's a huge bonus — you'll feel better in yourself, body and soul — livelier, more confident, more loving of yourself and your partner. Do keep your health at optimum levels. For more details see chapter 7 but regularly check the following basics are in place.

Daily exercise

Daily exercise builds muscle tone which makes you feel fit and look good too, all of which is good for your self-image and thus confidence in bed. Being active encourages good circulation which helps grow the network of capillaries to your clitoris, V spot and vulva and which gives you energy. It also releases hormones, such as adrenalin, which give you even more energy, and endorphins, which make you feel happy and loving. So walk, swim, dance, play tennis – do whatever you enjoy, but *do* make sure you're active.

Eat well

On holiday you eat lots of natural aphrodisiacs – olive oil and salads, fresh vegetables, garlic, fish and other protein. Passion needs feeding with a good mix of nutrients and vitamins. Give your body what it needs to feel fantastic and you'll feel super sexy as a result.

Sorry to be boring, but don't drink much alcohol before you make love. I know you may drink more than usual on holiday and still make love a lot, but if you think about it, you probably make love during your afternoon siesta on holiday or in the gap between the last swim of the afternoon and going out for dinner. Alcohol, contrary to popular opinion, is not an aphrodisiac – it might make you feel sexy initially, but it soon becomes a downer as far as sustained desire and arousal are concerned. Best avoided, other than a glass of wine, if you're going to make love.

Get outside in the fresh air and the light

We need sunlight for a range of health benefits. Obviously make sure you don't overdose – wear a sun hat, sunglasses when the light's glaring and good suncream and make certain you don't burn. But try to get at least half an hour of light outside, even in the winter. As well as giving you physical benefits, it will lift your mood and prevent you suffering from SAD – seasonal affective disorder – and the lowered sex drive, which is one of its symptoms.

Share time together whenever possible

On holiday you enjoy yourselves together and that builds a rapport that makes you desire each other sexually too. Why not do more together at home – live in the light together – don't be so solitary – go for a run, the two of you, rather than pounding the pavements alone, or walk to the pool to swim, or do whatever sport or outdoor activity you both enjoy.

Indoors, too, set some time aside to be together with nothing else to do but make love. Yes you CAN arrange it. Your sex life is worth it.

Conflict and rows

One of the most common traits of a relationship to cause anorgasmia is the tendency to react to differences and conflicts — which, let's face it, we're bound to have — with sarcasm, squabbling and/or rows or, even more perniciously, by blanking each other. But while the media often portrays rows or cold, steely silences as being intensely arousing, this scenario is rare in real life. Usually the truth is the exact opposite: conflict and anger are a turn-off. And when you do next make love, you're unlikely to have an orgasm unless you've said sorry and resolved any issues. Tension that's still simmering or has been buried stifles orgasmability, maybe because the hormones released in anger and resentment prevent the production of the feel-good ones that enable or assist orgasm, or because you simply can't get into an orgasmic mindset when you're still angry, consciously or subconsciously, with your partner. Or it can be because you're unwilling to let go to orgasm because you're damned if you're going to give him the power to give you pleasure.

Conflict between you may not be as open as a row. Perhaps you never or rarely squabble, but know that you disagree about many things and it makes you edgy or you sense that he is edgy with you. Or does one of you cope with the other's disagreeability by ignoring them, freezing them out or presuming the moral high ground? Or by subtle attacks, passive-aggressively, while pretending to be innocently sweet and nice to them? Any such discord and the ongoing circle of resentment, however low-key, can be all it takes to put the blocks on orgasm.

As an agony aunt and therapist, I spend a lot of time advising couples how to manage conflict resolution. It has a vital place in *every* relationship. In response to a difference of opinion you both look at the other's point of view, then work out the best way to address the problem or find a compromise that both of you can live with.

This can work well. But if you are in a relationship where differences are stopping you from enjoying sex right the way through to an orgasmic finish, it's my experience that you need to look beneath the specific differences themselves and get to the heart of your mutual attitude to each other's individuality and independence.

So often, we try to change this person we once loved more than anyone else. Some people – women and men – do this immediately when they get to know someone. Most couples, though, enjoy an in-love period where they feel amazingly similar in likes and dislikes, interests and viewpoints. During this mutual admiration time they don't row – they've nothing to row about because they're so alike. But as soon as reality dawns, as it always does, they see that they do have differences and don't think the same about a lot of things. And, boy oh boy, do some couples at this stage try to change each other, desperate to restore the sense of being as one.

He changed: Carry's story

I was horrified when I realised that Carl wasn't the sweet man who agreed with everything I said and didn't want to do the same things I did. He'd come out with the stupidest ideas and we'd argue and argue. He said it was me that was difficult and that I'd changed. Suddenly, he didn't want to make love to me as much, and when we did, he'd take ages to come. I found I'd get bored when we were having sex, and cross because I couldn't speed it up for him. I was resentful that I'd stopped having orgasms, but didn't realise that it wasn't just that our lovemaking had deteriorated in style – I was actually so angry at him for not being the man I thought he was that there was no way I was going to let him think he could give me an orgasm.

Carl wouldn't join Carry for counselling, but she relayed to him what we discussed: the need to see each other as having completely separate identities, with bad as well as good characteristics. We all have dark as well as light sides to our personalities. Recognising your partner isn't as perfect as you thought doesn't mean that you have to split up and look for someone who is perfect. You'll never find that person – they don't exist! It means it's time to accept them for who they really are, including all the things you don't care for much as well as the many aspects you do love. And then to let affection and love come back into your relationship – replacing hostile reactions to annoying traits with understanding or, at least, tolerance. Humour helps a lot. If you can gently tease each other about your respective faults, it goes a long way to getting them into perspective in your loving relationship as a whole, allowing you to appreciate all the things you do like about each other.

Then you're building a fundamental trust – that you're mutually appreciative and loving for real and not because of a romantic mirage; and compatibility and rapport have a chance to grow and blossom. These things are not always spontaneous in a relationship – they are usually brought into being and nurtured by thinking lovingly and caringly about each other and day by day deciding you want to be with each other, whatever else happens in your lives. Interestingly, the more mutually tolerant and appreciative a couple is, so that both feel they are loved 'warts and all', the more likely we are to tone down or rid ourselves of our bad points of our own volition.

Be nice to one another: Carry's story

It was so simple – but that's not to say easy! It horrified me how many times we both had to bite our tongues from put-downs like, 'Don't be so stupid,' or 'That's rubbish.' And for me, from nagging him to do what I wanted him to do. He realised how he was baulking from doing certain chores because he didn't want to be a yes-man. It took time but we gradually learnt to be a team while encouraging each other's independence too. We're still working on it – I guess we'll always have to. As a result, we stopped feeling selfish, which was the rut we had got into, and we began enjoying each other's bodies again and we just found ourselves loving sex again – and each other. Instead of waiting impatiently for Carl to come, I've cottoned on that I can let go and climax, and then have more orgasms. This turns him on and he usually comes much more quickly now – but if it does take a while, it's no problem because I'm enjoying myself anyway.

The orgasm-inhibiting habit of criticism

Often women tell me a negative criticism by their partner while having sex stopped them from climaxing. Not only did it stop them climaxing during that lovemaking session, for most it meant an ongoing disruption of their enjoyment of sex generally and for many a persistent difficulty in letting go to orgasm. And it caused some to lose desire for their partner completely.

A criticism like this doesn't mean he doesn't like having sex with you – it's just this one thing. You might, for instance, be squeezing him too roughly, and need to tone it down. Fine – do so. What I would say to him, though, is that if there's another instance where you're doing something that he doesn't like, instead of telling you what you are doing wrong, he should guide you gently to doing instead what will feel good. And agree that you'll both only ever say 'no' or 'don't do that' if the other refuses to listen and follow your guidance.

His criticism put me off: Sarah's story

We were having a fantastic time in bed, or at least I was and I thought he was too, and then he said, 'I wish you'd shut up – I can't bear it when you use language like that.' I know I can be mouthy when I'm getting very aroused but my previous partner said it turned him on and it never occurred to me that Dave wouldn't like it. It put me right off and I didn't come. He knew exactly why and apologised for having been so blunt but afterwards I said, 'Hey, I just wished you'd let me know in a gentler way – like telling me at a less vulnerable time that you find me most sexy when I'm quiet and that it bothers you when women swear, especially during lovemaking.' He saw the sense of that and since then we've listened to each other more carefully, reading between the lines – this way anything that could cause a problem is dealt with agreeably without causing offence or spoiling lovemaking.

But what if your partner has criticised you unreasonably for something that doesn't need to be changed or can't be? Then it smacks of another kind of the passive-aggression we mentioned above – they're using a mean comment to get at you for something else that's bugging them, which they haven't got the nerve to discuss.

He criticised my body: Angela's story

My last partner casually mentioned, as he gave my breasts a supposedly loving caress, that I'm 'pretty well totally flat-chested.' I was terribly upset. Hurt, first of all, then anxious that I looked awful to the point of thinking maybe I should have a boob job, then furious with him for being so cruel. After that I couldn't bring myself to make love to him. It finished it for me. When I told him the relationship was over, he told a friend he couldn't stand going out with a woman who had a powerful career and earned so much more than him. I realised that's what his spiteful comment was about. He was mad at me for something I couldn't help – his personal insecurity and envy. He didn't dare say this to my face so he punished me by criticising my body.

It takes two to make or mend a relationship, and perhaps if Angela had known how her partner felt, she could have helped him appreciate his own work and develop his self-esteem to a level where he was fine about her career, however different from his. And perhaps she could have looked out for any arrogance or inferred criticism of his earning power on her part and been more sensitive. Everything has worked out for her now – she met a man who was delighted to have a career-minded partner and who thinks her breasts are perfect just the way they are. Vitally, they are both comfortable discussing anything that has or may have an effect on their relationship.

Intimacy and trust

Intimacy and trust go hand-in-hand and, in a long-term relationship, form a necessary foundation for orgasms. Sure, the excitement born of challenge or lust early in a relationship can trigger easy orgasms. But sooner or later, the fact a man won't fully commit to you ceases to sexually excite you, and lust loses its lustre. Long term, if you don't trust your partner, you'll start holding something of yourself back, effectively detaching yourself from him. That something could be your willingness to orgasm with him or could cause you to withdraw it. Such holding back is a natural instinct of pride or self-preservation, depending where you are with your self-esteem.

If your long-term relationship is monogamous by agreement, to become and remain truly intimate you need to believe your partner when he says he loves you and is faithful to you, and it needs to be true, and believed by him, when you tell him the same. Otherwise there will be an element of dishonesty lurking between you which will preclude intimacy. And usually when intimacy is out of the picture so, for the woman, is orgasm.

I didn't trust him after the affair: Beth's story

I imagined him telling her she was very special and giving her the impression he might leave me. That's what people do, isn't it, when they start an affair? And I kept thinking, if he's done it once, he'll have another one. Although our lovemaking was fantastic, better than ever, I completely lost the knack of climaxing. I just couldn't get myself over the brink, even if I masturbated. We went to therapy together and our counsellor suggested that I should pretend to believe him when he said he loved me and wanted to be faithful. So I tried, and found it made me feel wonderful – like falling in love with him all over again. So then I thought, well I've got a lot to gain by believing him for real – it was a matter of deciding to trust him. It seems to me that no one can know for sure whether they or their partner will be true forever. But the future is the future. All we can do is live in the present and make it as good as we can. So I trust him and it's given a depth to our relationship. We're closer than we've ever been and it's as though this emotional intimacy nurtures the intimacy of orgasms because I started having them again as soon as I stopped resisting his pledge to be faithful.

Beth was fortunate to have that suggestion from her counsellor and to be willing to try it. Yes, trusting a partner and allowing intimacy to grow between you is a leap of faith, especially if they've let you down once, but it's well worth it. Your trust will encourage them to honour your belief and be true to you. And even if the relationship doesn't work out forever, in the meantime you'll enjoy being with them and discover or resume orgasmic sex.

Rapport

When physical and emotional intimacy combine, it smooths the way for you to create a rapport in all facets of your life together and to understand what drives you individually.

Being familiar with each other's personalities in all the various emotional and practical aspects makes hostile clashes far less likely and when you do have one, the mutual understanding will speed you through. Remembering and renewing your wish to be together on a daily basis will also help you ride the ups and downs of life and your interaction.

This very pragmatic approach to getting on well on a day-to-day basis will inevitably, if it's what you want, deepen and expand your physical bond. The gentleness between you, the compassion, the affection and the understanding will all help create an alchemy of sensual sexuality.

And if you're going to have sex with the same person, long term, it had better be great, hadn't it? That doesn't mean it has to be athletic or inventive or even varied — great sex is mutually extremely enjoyable sex. It's a huge blessing of life and a relationship and, without it, one of you will get bored or resentful and then you could be on a downward spiral back to mistrust.

Great sex doesn't have to be orgasmic, of course. But if climax is possible for you, then why miss out on something that's so enjoyable and so good for your relationship, too? It seems to me it's worth polishing all the facets of your relationship to help enable you to be easily, blissfully orgasmic.

Does your social life have anything to do with being orgasmic?

The part of your relationship between you and your partner that's on display to your friends will influence their impression of how well you get on and how happy you are together. All of this will affect their attitude to you, your partner and your relationship, and their attitude in turn could influence you and your partner and thus perhaps even your relationship and orgasmability.

The energy we each produce is influenced by our mood, self-belief and the emotional climate between ourselves and others, especially our partner. When positive energy surrounds us it attracts the same back from our friends. Be negative and we magnetise negativity from others towards ourselves.

Friends are constantly taking in where you are with your sexual, sensual, emotional and general rapport with your partner. They'll respond accordingly, keeping in tune with what they're sensing. It's a bit like a dance of empathy, when the tone is positive or when negative of hostility. This effect can be ongoing. If the impression your friends receive is of a warm, loving connection between you and your partner, they'll refer to and treat you as a happily together couple. This will feel good to you both and encourage more appreciation. It will help make you feel sexually together too. It's nice to be in a relationship which seems to outsiders to be fulfilled. You'll be glad the impression is for real, and, feeling good about your rapport is the perfect foundation for great sex, including orgasms.

All we did was complain about each other: Sara's story

I'd make my friends laugh about our various disputes and I needed to offload, so it made me feel better and I'd do it more and more. So I laid it on thicker and thicker and I suppose to them John began to sound worse than he really is – he's actually quite a nice man, if I'm honest – it was just we were both so intolerant and rubbed each other up the wrong way. But my friends started to see him as a bit of an ogre. They'd advise me to stand up for myself and rallied round me protectively when John was with me. When we snapped at each other or rowed in front of them, which we were always doing, they'd automatically take my side. So I began to feel like a victim.

Then one day when I was with my friends and my mother happened to be there, she saw what was going on and stuck up for him. Afterwards she told me I was jolly lucky to have him and should try being nicer to him, and that it was disloyal to bad-mouth him to my friends. Mum said if I wasn't careful, he'd leave me and I suddenly knew she was right and it terrified me. Because I'd begun to believe the horrible persona of John that my friends and I had conjured up, I'd begun detaching myself from him on the sexual front too. Saying no to sex, most times, and making it clear I didn't really want to when we did. There was no way I was going to have an orgasm in those circumstances and, as this situation had been building for a long time, I must have gone without an orgasm for two years at least. It wasn't all my fault – he could be as nasty to me as I was to him. But when my mother made me face what we'd got ourselves into, I knew we had to do something radical or we'd break up.

Sara and John had a long talk and it turned out her worry was justified – he had been increasingly disheartened by their bickering and the way everyone seemed to think it was all his fault. Although he thought it was unfair, he didn't want to have to defend himself to anyone – and he knew he gave as good as he got anyway, so it wasn't any more Sara's fault than his. At a counsellor's suggestion, they made a list of promises and, at a reception to celebrate the renewal of their commitment to each other, pledged to keep them all.

They showed me the list:

1. I will tell you when I feel cross or hurt and we will explore the reason together.

2. I will not blame or shame you, even when I do think it's about you.

3. We will resolve any justified grievance either of us may have together or bridge any difference causing a problem.

4. I will not ever criticise you when we are with our friends or demean you in any way.

5. As much as possible, I will show my support for you and my belief in you.

6. When I disagree with you about something, I will show my respect for your right to your opinion.

7. I will not talk about you derogatorily behind your back or foster the impression that you are difficult to live with or that I am hard done by.

8. I will not use your characteristics to make myself appear in a better light.

9. I will not use our social life to score points off you.

10. I will treat your personal friends pleasantly and kindly and, even if they don't appeal to me, try to see what you like about them.

Can you create rapport?

This question has two parts – general rapport, the kind that makes living together a pleasure and enables friendship, and, in a long-term relationship, sexual rapport.

General rapport can certainly be helped to exist, and maintained, by conscious attention and effort. To illustrate this, people often get on well with members of their family who they might not have gelled with if, unrelated, they'd met as strangers elsewhere. Similarly, in the village where I live we've all become friends because we've been thrown together in a fairly remote community whereas had we not met here we probably wouldn't have connected in the same way, as we're all very different. Here we've made an effort to get to know and like each other and succeeded in creating a network of rapport between us in all kinds of emotional and practical ways.

Even when you don't spontaneously like someone on first meeting, or when you irritate the hell out of each other at some stage, it's often possible if one, or preferably both, of you pay attention to what's going on between you to change the negative interaction to positive and create or renew rapport.

A couple can do this too. It's about consciously taking an interest in each other, even when you may have become disinterested, and being nice, even when you don't feel like it. You know, we can usually come up with something positive to say if we try. I'm not talking about being sycophantic or creepy – but being like a warm, positive, kind, generous, interested and interesting human being to another. Look for the good in him.

Remember what you liked about him when you first met and were getting to know each other. It's still there for the seeing.

Sexual rapport can certainly be recreated and can, sometimes, be created from a blank canvas. To rediscover it, as above, remember how you used to feel. Really feel it again now, reliving it in your mind. Remember how you fancied him, loved his face, his body, his voice. How it felt when you were near him, touching him, making love. The desire, arousal and, if you used to have one, climax. Be there, in your mind, all over again. Now, when you look at him, see that same person. Imagine you are going to feel the same now as you did then. If the feelings don't start to come back, then invite them in by pretending. Pretend he's incredibly attractive to you and you want him to touch you, make love to you. Pretend, when you are making love, that you feel as you used to. Living the recreation of your attraction like this can make it real again.

I'd forgotten what attracted me to him in the first place: Gerri's story

I'd gone off my partner Will and thought we'd have to split up because, although we had a good life together, I didn't want to make love to him any more. There was no way I was going to climax, feeling like that, and the whole thing had become something I dreaded. Talking to a counsellor, I admitted that I'd always gone off men, however strong the initial attraction. She said that the chemical attraction always fades when you've been together for a while, sometimes completely, and that keeping attraction and desire for each other alive is all in the mind. As I liked Will so much and our relationship had so much going for it, I followed her suggestions, not thinking about my present feelings when I was with him but remembering and emulating how I felt at the beginning of our relationship. To my astonishment, it worked. He really turned me on, so much so that I climaxed for the first time in ages. I practised being very smoochy and affectionate with him whatever we were doing and he was so pleased he started being romantic and very loving towards me too, so we were acting like sweethearts. Well, we are. It isn't a sham at all – we really are. Thank goodness I didn't kick him out – I couldn't have a better partner and lover.

Doing things together, while I'm on the subject, is great for recreating rapport generally and sexually in a tired relationship. Kim and Nick had grown apart, so much so that they were wondering why they were still married. He'd gone off sex and she'd gone off trying to seduce him. She'd been anorgasmic for some time anyway.

Spending time together saved our relationship: Kim's story

It all changed when we started doing crosswords. Don't ask me why we did – neither of us had done them but one weekend it was pouring with rain and there was nothing on TV. We were reading through the weekend papers and I started doing the crossword, reading out the clues to him if I got stuck. We hadn't laughed so much together since we were at college, which is where we met. And when we did manage to make progress, it was so satisfying – but a kind of mutual satisfaction. I happened to laugh to a friend that it's brought us really close again to the extent that we're having great sex and I'm having orgasms, which is brilliant. Now 'doing a crossword' is a euphemism in our gang of friends for having it off together! Nick loves the teasing because it shows that everyone thinks we're a really sexy, loving couple – and we are.

It doesn't matter what you do together as long as it gets you laughing, makes you face challenges, however small, pushes you to follow each other's lead, makes you talk or be physically close, it will make you close as a couple – and being close as a couple is the prelude to great, orgasmic lovemaking. Laughter and play work the same way.

Mutual support

I was at a party some time ago and we were joined by a woman, Rennie, who arrived on her own. I didn't know her, but the others did and one of them asked where her partner was. 'His old dog died this morning,' she said, 'and he didn't feel like coming out.'

'I'm so sorry about the dog,' I said. 'You must be pretty cut up too?'

'It's sad,' she replied, 'but he was Mike's dog more than mine – and there's no point sitting at home feeling miserable.'

She looked and acted the opposite, confirming what I'd sensed as soon as she said she'd left him at home to grieve alone – their relationship was empty.

Dressed up to the nines, she quickly charmed another male guest and they spent the rest of the evening locked in conversation. I heard later they began an affair that night and almost immediately she left her old partner for the new one.

Months later I got to know – and like – Rennie. She confirmed what I'd since heard – that Mike's neglect and disdain had gradually suffocated her love for him. She didn't say as much, but it was clear that abandoning him to his grief was an accumulated reaction to years of his low-key but insidious emotional abuse.

His lack of support wore away my love: Rennie's story

I knew that you thought I was cold and heartless not staying at home with Mike that evening. But I couldn't take any more. He hadn't wanted sex for two years. Before then, I only did it because I felt I had to. I never had an orgasm with him. When I met Sam at that party, it was a head-on sexual attraction and there was no way I was going to ignore it. I climaxed with him for the first few weeks, but we were all wrong for each other in all kinds of practical ways. When the animal attraction faded, he didn't turn me on any more.

We only lasted a matter of weeks, to be honest. I had a few casual relationships after him but I still couldn't climax. I thought I never would – that I'd lost the ability forever.

Meanwhile I'd been sorting my life out – what I wanted to do deep inside me. I went to university as a mature student and then did further business training in management while working for a large local firm. I made an interesting, thoroughly enjoyable life on my own. So when I met Les, another macho alpha-male by reputation, I was a good match for him – not a bit like the 'yes' girl I'd been with Mike. We have a great relationship – very equal – and I've never been happier in bed. Either one of us can take the lead. Whatever we do, we're very together – and the sex is orgasmic in every sense of the word, always. We're careful not to mock each other, put each other down – you know how some couples do? If one of us tries that, the other will immediately point it out. We're determined not to let that kind of rot set in. We think about each other's feelings and are careful not to hurt each other. He's kind to me and that allows me to be girlie and sweet – sometimes anyway! – without the fear that he'll take advantage and start bossing me about like Mike did. He's not frightened of me but I'm not a pushover, either, whereas in hindsight I think Mike was both those things – frightened of me but despising me at the same time. We never bully each other and we always do our best to be support- ive and loyal. If he's suffering, I'm there for him and I always will be. He's the same with me. We're a proper couple – a team.

Mutual support, in small and large ways, is part of the fabric, part of the balance of a mutually nourishing rela- tionship. We need to know our partner's there with us, emotionally, every step of the way. It's fundamental to our orgasmability in a long-term relationship. It's about trust and intimacy and balance. Without it, all these fall by the wayside.

Work-life balance

Happiness for you and your partner is much about hav- ing a comfortable balance between careers, domestic work, personal interests and quality time together and with your family.

For centuries the custom for most marriages was for the woman to assume a stereotypical feminine role and the man a masculine one. She did emotions, he – if he admitted he had them – didn't show them. Some couples still follow this pattern and where it suits both partners, it can still work well. But increasingly we're expected to be pretty much equally capable in all aspects of our life together. We hear a lot about 'new' men but there are new types of women too. These days few women exclusively look after the domestic needs of their children and husband; instead, we want a job we can enjoy, financial and social independence and to manage our lives the way we want. We realise that while being totally feminine, we can shoulder the traditionally 'masculine' jobs if we wish, and men know that their intrinsic masculinity includes the ability to take on roles previously thought of as 'feminine' – they want to help bring up their children, be well in touch with their emotions and enjoy deep, mutually understanding intimacy with their partner.

A friend of mine, Jeff, said, 'It's about yin and yang really, isn't it? We are all a mixture of so-called masculine and feminine traits. Ideally, when these are well balanced in each person and in a relationship, this translates as equality. Of course we're different in many ways and that's fantastic – it would be pretty boring otherwise. But as different as a couple are, they should ideally be equal.'

Thank goodness, we are free today to explore and discover our own particular balance. But because our roles have changed so much and so quickly over the past few decades, we are still adjusting, and many of us are finding it difficult to adapt. Not everyone finds role adjustment or reversal easy and when power struggles ensue, they can scupper desire, arousal and orgasms.

The solution is to see the benefits of balance as an individual and equality as a couple, rather than bemoaning the loss of the old standards. Yes, they had their good points, but potentially the new roles we're still working out and adjusting too have so much more going for them.

Sexually, this has huge implications. Free to enjoy our sexuality and sex life autonomously rather than at our partner's discretion, we stand to gain far more insight and understanding of the orgasmic path from desire through arousal to climax itself. Enjoying sex is nothing new, of course, but in the past women were made to believe by the male-dominated culture that it was only acceptable to do so within a marriage. Today women in the West are able to be in touch with their sexuality throughout their teenage and adult lives – surely the best possible foundation for finding fulfilment sexually and being orgasmic in the most complete sense.

I've changed my way of thinking: Jeff's story

My first wife stayed at home with our children just as our mothers did with us – we assumed it was the right thing to do. But she missed her career and disliked having to make do on my salary. To my shame, when she tried to tell me about her feelings, I remember shouting at her, 'Why can't you be a normal woman and just enjoy looking after the kids and me?' After that she went off sex, big time, and even when I did persuade her to make love, she no longer climaxed. I thought she'd simply fallen out of love with me. I realise now that however much she loved us, she had so many other aspects to her personality, and she felt her whole balance was being compromised, stuck at home. That unbalanced our relationship – it seems so obvious to me now but at the time we just resented each other, felt trapped and eventually the only way forward was to break out of the trap by getting divorced.

My new partner and I take the time to help each other through whatever ups and downs and imbalances we're facing. I don't feel I have to be macho all the time – I can cry and tell her about my fears. And I respect her ability in all kinds of things that I couldn't have coped with from my first wife as I'd have been jealous or insecure. Sue and I know we can be who we are – we never have to pretend. I guess it reflects in our sex life. Because there's no resentment or hidden agenda in our individual personalities and life together, when we make love, we can concentrate on the pleasure, pure and simple. If she ever had problems climaxing, we'd have to find out why and put it right – but there are certainly no worries on that front now.

Women today like Sue are less likely than their foremothers to lay the responsibility for their orgasms solely on their partner or relationship. By reading this book, you're showing your strong sense of self-esteem and your belief in yourself to nurture your sexuality.

One of the blessings of finding a good balance with a partner who is, like you, well balanced or working on it, is the comfortableness of lovemaking. You fall into place together like two malleable pieces in a jigsaw. It's no big deal to make time and take time, you just do so, often, because sex feels apt, and wholesome, and when you orgasm — as you will find you begin to — it's a sign that the balance is for those moments in perfect harmony and you let go to the magic, full of gladness for the joy.

Finding the perfect balance: Sandra's story

Orgasm feels to me like our respective yin and yang and our relationship has met in the middle of the triangle and fused together to make the sweetest energy imaginable. It's only happened for me since I've found my own inner balance and now it's there with Rob. I guess we'll always keep it in mind. It's like finding gold but it's gold that's there, potentially, in every person and every relationship. Tell your readers it's well worth finding — it did it for me!

Attraction

What is it that attracts you to someone? Have you felt the instant kind of attraction — real eyes across the room stuff? If so, was it their looks or their body that appealed to you? Or are you a slow burner type of person, needing to get to know a potential partner before attraction starts to build?

Experiencing intense attraction can doubtlessly be a great help to being orgasmic. When you patently want someone very physically, it jumps you straight into desire and up the arousal curve in leaps and bounds and probably into spontaneous climax. There's no need for practising technique or fantasising or removing blocks of any kind – you'll just be there in a whoosh of desire and pleasure and satisfaction.

This feeling is fantastic – and you can understand why people get hooked on it. But if that kind of animal attraction is going to last, it has to eventually be backed up with a real liking and love for each other and, yes, good technique. Because even the best sex in the world can become, though I hate to say it, samey if not boring.

And, of course, the things that attracted you and your partner to each other may not endure automatically. If you're thinking, 'My partner used to be attractive but he's let himself go,' or if you've let yourself go and feel unattractive, it's not going to do much for your sex life.

We both stopped caring: Ling's story

When we first starting going out, we were a great-looking couple. Although Tim couldn't care less about fashion he made an effort to dress well and I wouldn't have dreamt of going out in anything scruffy or without a face of make-up. A few years later I no longer had to look smart for the office as I worked from home to be with our two kids, so it was easiest to wear old clothes in the daytime, as it didn't matter if they got grubby or covered in paint or play dough. For a while I'd change once the kids were in bed, but then once or twice I didn't get round to it, and soon I never bothered. Tim followed suit and started changing into an old tracksuit when he got home – and pretty soon we stopped flirting and snogging and completely stopped fancying each other.

It wasn't just that we took your advice to start making an effort to look nice for each other that revived our sex life, but it made a big difference. Thinking it through, it wasn't the clothes and the fact we looked nice again, though, of course, that made us feel good about ourselves and each other. It was the fact that I was making an effort for him and he for me – that was a surprising turn-on, and also that it made us start paying attention to each other again. Like he'd say to me, once I'd changed into something fresh and put a bit of make-up on,

'Hey, you look nice, come here for a cuddle.' We became very aware of each other physically again. The old attraction was still there – by neglecting it, we'd sent it into hibernation, that was all. We'll always keep it awake from now on. The combination of being relaxed together and pleasantly, sexily aware of each other's appearance has also, somehow, made me orgasmic – something I'd struggled for years before with no luck.

This can work almost in the same way if you never had an intense sexual attraction or even any at all, but you do need to like their face and body and being very close emotionally and, especially, physically.

One friend of mine puts it down to this: 'You've got to like their smell. If you can kiss their skin, say, on their arm, and breathe in their body scent and you just love it, that's the foundation of a sexual attraction. I adore my partner's scent – so much so that if he's away, I'll keep a shirt he's worn back from the wash and bury my face in it just to smell him. And don't laugh but I love kissing his armpits – the smell of his fresh sweat really turns me on.'

I think she's right that liking someone's body scent is an important element of attraction, though I'd add

pheromones – the scent around us that we don't consciously pick up on but which is nevertheless very
important to sexual attraction.

So if you like a guy and like the smell of him – and
I'm talking about the natural scent of his skin, sweat
and breath – that's the basic foundation on which you
may be able to create attraction if you don't immediately
feel it. Ideally, build emotional and practical rapport
first. That is, become friends, discover a mutual spiri-
tual understanding if possible, have fun doing things
together and socialising. Then use your mind, as above,
to imagine how it would feel to be strongly attracted to
him and go on from there.

Attraction is precious – look after it.

Chapter 7

Health and Well-Being

We need to feel okay physically to enjoy an active, orgasmic sex life. That's not to say that ill-health precludes great sex – in fact, it can, by encouraging you to think how you're going to get round the difficulties your condition presents, help you have better pleasure than ever.

But you do need to review and manage health problems to allow you to continue to make love to yourself or with your partner; otherwise they can loom all too large and block desire, arousal and climax at any stage.

So check out possible difficulties and learn how you can resolve them or navigate around them when making love.

Painful sex

If it hurts when you have foreplay or intercourse, it's bound to put you off and make orgasm unlikely. The good news is that this problem can often be addressed with self-help techniques as described below, but do see your doctor first to check a medical condition isn't causing the problem.

Tightness and vaginismus

Vaginismus is the tendency to have a vaginal muscle spasm that feels as though it 'locks' the entrance to the vagina. It often happens to young women who are having sex for the first time and are very nervous. However, it can also happen for other reasons, such as after experiencing sex that was painful, following an emotional or physical trauma such as a miscarriage, painful birthing, perhaps with an episiotomy, or sexual abuse. Vaginal tightness can occur simply if you are very tired, don't want sex for any reason, are post-menopausal or have been torn during childbirth or had a too severe repair after an episiotomy. Vaginismus and tightness can make penetration seem impossible or very difficult and if your partner forces his way inside you with his fingers or penis, it will hurt a lot. With the memory of this pain added to the nervousness, there's no way future attempts are going to get easier without your self-help.

What you can do

Seek treatment for any condition likely to cause pain. Then gradually practise getting yourself ready for and used to penetration by taking time every day to pleasure yourself (see chapter 3).

Here are two exercises that can help prepare and relax your vagina.

Preparing for intercourse

Exercise 1

Step 1: When you're in bed, use plenty of lubricant and practise inserting a finger in your vagina.

Step 2: Once you're comfortable with this, try two fingers. Keeping them still, focus on how this feels. Breathe slowly and deeply, relaxing every part of your body.

Step 3: When you're comfortable, gently widen your fingers, feeling how much scope your vagina has. It helps to remember that it's designed to expand.

Exercise 2

Step 1: When you're in a warm bath, a useful exercise is
to lie with your back flat on the bottom of the bath
with your feet drawn up towards your hips.

Step 2: Now insert a finger and hold the vaginal
entrance open just a little, allowing some water to
flow inside you. Relax and allow the muscles around
your vagina to relax. You'll feel your vagina balloon
out slightly.

Step 3: Now withdraw your finger and express the water
by bearing down (as though trying to urinate).

Step 4: Do the exercise again, this time flexing your PC
muscle against your finger before expelling the water
as before.

Step 5: Keep doing this a few times to familiarise yourself with the flexibility of your vagina and how to
relax it easily (it's a good way of exercising your PC
muscle too!).

When you can do this exercise comfortably, try doing it
when you're masturbating. Take plenty of time to get

seriously aroused first. Then see how much easier it is than when you were doing it 'cold'. If you have a partner, do the exercise when you're extremely aroused through petting and once you have verified that your vaginal entrance is stretchy and ready, guide him in (see chapter 5). The key, as ever, is being really aroused and using lots of lubricant.

Clinical therapy
When I was training in psychosexual therapy, during clinical attendance I watched the physician, a specialist in psychosexual therapy, treat cases of vaginismus. Even though the patients were unaroused and understandably tense, after applying lubricant, he would gently insert a small circumference dilator – usually much to the client's amazement that he was able to do so easily and it didn't hurt. At subsequent appointments he'd repeat the exercise with the second and third sizes. Gentleness, good lubrication and extreme care made what each woman thought impossible pain-free and easy. Finally he'd ask them to go home and practise with their fingers and, once fully comfortable with their ability to do this, have sex with their partner and guide his penis inside them.

The self-help route is equally doable and successful. However if you have deep-seated mental or emotional issues that make it difficult for you to relax and become comfortably accustomed to your vagina's stretchability, psychosexual therapy may be helpful in getting you through this.

A further note on post-menopausal tightness
After the menopause the vagina tends to lose its natural capacity for stretchiness if we don't have regular sex. Many women find that the above exercises often gradually encourage renewed flexibility so that you can have comfortable intercourse once more. If not, explain to your partner that it's just not practical any more so that he knows it's not that you've gone off him and the idea of intercourse as such. Sex without intercourse is hugely enjoyable and if you're both having plenty of pleasure through manual and/or oral sex, you can both be amply satisfied and fulfilled. But don't just say no to intercourse – do explain to him what's happened.

Vaginal tear during childbirth or episiotomy repair

After either a vaginal tear during childbirth or episiotomy repair it will take at least several weeks and possibly months to heal sufficiently for intercourse. Meanwhile, if you want to make love, ask your partner to avoid the area around your vaginal entrance and concentrate instead on the clitoral area – that is the clitoral hood, shaft and V spot (see chapter 5). If a couple of months after an episiotomy repair it's still too sore for pleasurable touch – let alone intercourse – consult your GP or gynaecologist. It may be that you need another procedure to widen the opening sufficiently to allow comfortable, pleasurable intercourse once more.

Medical conditions
There are many other reasons why you may be experiencing pain during intercourse. This could be due to a vaginal infection, viral warts or herpes, inflamed cervix or other cervical problem, bladder irritation or pelvic inflammatory disease, ovarian cyst, a womb polyp or a fibroid in the cervix, prolapse, ovary or womb cancer, irritable bowel or endometriosis. Scar tissue at the top of the vagina after a hysterectomy could also cause intercourse to be painful.

Or perhaps you may have an allergy or sensitivity to something you're using. This could be from a particular make of condom, spermicide or lubricant. It could even be a product you're using in the bath or the laundry.

A painful skin sensitivity was the problem: Beth's story

I'd try to let him have intercourse but it was so uncomfortable there was no way I could have an orgasm – all I thought about was the pain. The doctor suggested I stopped using bubble bath or shower gel and to just wash with a pure soap, rinsing the area once a day with slightly salty water. He also recommended using gentle soap flakes to wash my knickers in case detergent was the culprit. The problem disappeared almost immediately so I guess I'd had some kind of allergic reaction.

Never be coerced into intercourse you believe will be painful. The above familiarisation and stretching exercise will reassure you that you are ready for and able to have intercourse – only then, go ahead. It's just not worth risking or tolerating pain – it will put you off sex and do nothing for your orgasmability. It's well worth waiting as you practise until you welcome intercourse again and can fully relax and enjoy it, absolutely pain-free.

Remember too that if you're experiencing any kind of pain during intercourse only your doctor can give you a correct diagnosis, so it's important that you consult him or her if pain persists.

Managing pain caused by illness or disability
Chronic pain doesn't have to inhibit the enjoyment of sex but all too often it does put us off the idea completely. And if we do go ahead, it preys on the mind so much that an orgasm is out of the question.

The good news is that sexual pleasure and orgasm are natural painkillers if we have the mindset and ability to enjoy them. But sometimes we simply haven't — it depends on the pain, our mood and how our energy levels are affecting us. Migraine, for instance, can make some sufferers feel so wretched that any activity, let alone sex, is intolerable. Some people find that even if they feel pretty dreadful, sex can relieve the pain and other symptoms and even heal them completely. It can depend on the stage of the migraine too — if one is just beginning, the mood lift, relaxation and circulation boost that sex and orgasm produce have been known to dissolve the attack before it has a chance to set in.

Forcing yourself to have sex or pushing for an orgasm against your better judgement isn't a good idea. Only ever make love to yourself or with a partner when *you* want to, or when you perhaps don't feel well but sense that sexual pleasure will make you feel better emotionally by taking your mind off the pain or discomfort and perhaps giving you some physical relief from it too.

So if you have an illness or condition that causes recurrent or chronic pain or discomfort, but would like to be able to enjoy an orgasmic sex life anyway, it's important to know yourself, your illness and the nature of the hurt you feel and learn what you can do to manage it. There's a brilliant book that advises comprehensively on managing pain called *Manage Your Pain*, which is listed in Useful Resources (see page 242).

When sex is difficult because a disability makes movement or pressure painful or awkward, experiment very gently, stopping immediately if you experience discomfort.

Spend some time alone finding a position to lie or sit in that's most comfortable for you. With your partner, have fun working out how you can fit together so that each of you feels relaxed and comfortable. If this seems impossible, remember you can have great pleasure taking turns to make love to each other rather than trying to move your bodies together in sync. And remember, when it's your turn to lie back and concentrate on the sensations and waves of pleasure, guide him gently to the touch you prefer if he's not sure (see chapter 5).

For further advice, discuss the positions for lovemaking likely to be best for you with your physiotherapist.

Dryness

If we don't lubricate naturally, it's easy to think we're somehow lacking in sexiness and this does nothing for our libido and orgasmability. Actually, it has nothing to do with how highly sexed we are – a whole gamut of things affect lubrication and many women, however feminine and sexy they are, simply don't produce much of the stuff.

Without treatment, dryness makes intercourse decidedly uncomfortable and even vulval and clitoral pleasuring with no penetration benefits from the feeling of suppleness and silkiness that lubrication provides.

So if your vagina has a tendency not to produce enough lubrication, identify the cause and remedy it if possible. If you are one of many women who simply don't produce enough, buy lubricant regularly and slather it on whenever you masturbate or make love with a partner.

Dryness can be caused by any number of psychological issues, ranging from self-esteem to depression. See the relevant sections or a counsellor to help identify and get to the heart of any issues upsetting you so that you can resolve them. Many illnesses and medications have dryness as a possible side effect and if this is a possibility for you, it's best to consult your doctor. Hormone fluctuations, for instance, at certain times of your monthly cycle, or in and after the menopause, are probably the most common cause of vaginal dryness.

Dryness doesn't necessarily mean you aren't aroused and won't have orgasms, it doesn't mean you're not sexy and it doesn't mean you or your partner aren't pleasuring you right or enough, but if you worry about any of these, it could put you off getting aroused or having an orgasm. So remember that some of us just don't lubricate naturally, however great our desire or arousal or however many orgasms we have. But, yes, being well lubricated is sexy because it feels good and greatly increases sexual pleasure and hence orgasms, too, so apply heaps of lube and re-apply often and then it won't matter a bit whether you make any yourself or not.

Hormone balance

Don't let anyone tell you hormones don't disrupt your libido and orgasmability – they surely can. Being aware of any regular waves of desire can be very useful in making the most of our sex drive and dealing constructively with unsettled phases can help avoid or soothe libido and arousal problems.

Taking advantage of your natural cycle

Get to know your own cycle and make the most of the days you're ovulating to make love, as this is the time when you'll probably feel your sexiest and thus get aroused and climax most easily.

With some forms of the pill, you won't ovulate but your hormones will form a pattern anyway and it's quite likely you'll feel particularly sexy for a few days mid-cycle. If so, use those feelings and be inspired to make love – it may well be the most compatible time to start having orgasms.

Get to know your cycle: Gina's story

I have a libido surge about halfway through my cycle, lasting for a few days when I'm ovulating. I'll feel really, really sexy and become more easily orgasmic than usual and, although I'm never desperate for sex like some women, I do feel as though I need an orgasm each day at least during those few days.

Just before and during a period

Just before our period many of us experience premenstrual tension, as this is when hormones tend to fluctuate more dramatically than at any other time of the month. If you tend to slump emotionally, you may not feel like sex at all and that's fine. But it's worth trying to make love at least once at this time, if you never have, to see if you're one of the women who finds that once they get through the barrier of their mood, they are surprisingly receptive to pleasure. Remember intercourse and oral sex, if you don't fancy them at this time of the month, aren't necessary – you can have a great time with manual clitoral and V spot touch alone. If you have stomach ache or cramps, an orgasm will make you oblivious to them for a few blissful seconds and you may well find them considerably eased afterwards.

Pregnancy

Again, don't make assumptions about how you ought or ought not to feel when you're pregnant. Some women go off sex at some time during their pregnancy, especially during the early months if they experience nausea, and at the end of their pregnancy if they feel uncomfortably huge. Follow your doctor's advice on whether it's okay for you to have sex, and if the answer's yes, I suggest giving it a try as you may find it's very pleasurable.

Many women feel exceptionally feminine during pregnancy and their libido soars. If you don't want to have intercourse or it's uncomfortable or unpractical because of your shape, both manual and oral sex are brilliant alternatives.

After giving birth

The medical advice is to wait until your post-natal check (usually six weeks after the birth) before having intercourse and I'd emphasise the words *at least*. If you were torn during delivery or had an episiotomy, the tissues within the vagina and around the opening will need plenty of time to recover from their trauma and it may take longer than six weeks to fully heal. And until they do, there's no way you'll be ready for intercourse. This doesn't mean you can't have sex through non-penetrative manual or oral touch. But obviously it's essential to be very, very careful not to do anything that will affect the soreness in or around your vaginal opening so be very gentle and make sure your partner realises he needs to be too. Listen to your body and mind – be content to wait for desire to return or resurge and as it does, notice and encourage it with love, erotic thoughts and fantasies.

Breastfeeding may or may not make you feel sexy. If you find breastfeeding turns you on sexually, enjoy and 'hold' the feeling and once your baby goes to sleep, make love to yourself or with your partner – you may find yourself surprisingly orgasmic.

Post-natal depression
Once again, never force yourself or be coerced into having sex you don't want. But do encourage yourself to try giving it a go – on your own or with your partner – as the feel-good hormones sexual pleasure and orgasm release will lift your depression at least in the moment and possibly have a long-lasting effect.

Getting through the post-natal blues: Kiely's story

Be very gentle and kind to yourself generally and get as much support and help as possible from your health visitor, doctor, family, friends and neighbours. Remember most people are only too glad to have the opportunity to help but don't like to 'interfere' unasked – so don't hesitate to ask them. Remember, too, that most people realise that it's often difficult being a new mum and are aware of the likelihood of post-natal depression and will be sympathetic and keen to be useful. On the sexual front, don't be even more depressed if you've lost your sex drive completely – most of us in our group of new mums did for a while. My good news is that I was so pleased when I stopped being depressed and at long last felt sexy again, I had my first orgasm ever. It was like my body giving me a huge hug and it blew away the last cobwebs of depression completely.

Menopause and other potential time for hormone disruption

Even after the menopause, once your hormones have settled down again, you may experience a monthly surge when sex is on your mind more than usual and you spontaneously want sex. You may even get aroused and climax more quickly and with less effort than usual.

Listen to your body: Claire's story

I've only recently started having orgasms and when I'm having sex with my partner, it usually takes about half an hour. But yesterday I was alone in the house and was feeling a bit horny and I realised I fancied giving myself an orgasm. I didn't have much time so assumed it was unlikely I'd be able to, but I went ahead anyway. I focused exclusively on my V spot and Mount of Venus, pressing, pulsing and pausing like you'd suggested and almost immediately started to get aroused. Astonishingly, I realised after what seemed like a couple of minutes, and was certainly no more than five, that I was getting that 'coming up to brink' feeling. I panicked for a moment, scared of losing it, but told myself that, no matter, I should just enjoy whatever happens. I paused and counted to three and then pressed gently again, and it just happened completely effortlessly – the best orgasm I've ever had. If I hadn't listened to that initial 'I fancy an orgasm feeling', I might have missed it!

Take notice of how you feel and if you are feeling sexy and generally good about yourself, then take advantage of it and have sex. Orgasms are always easiest when we feel vibrant. Some people are very susceptible to seasonal changes in the weather and heavy air pressure at any time. Daylight and sunshine boost some of the feel-good vitamins and, in turn, help hormone production and balance.

Wherever you are on your life path, be aware of how you are responding to the surrounding world and conditions and of your body's natural cycles and rhythms.

During the menopause, and possibly at times of illness or when you're not eating as well as usual, your hormones may be in a state of corresponding adjustment.

My libido changed: Lin's story

I don't know where my libido went when I was going through the menopause. I thought it had died and I'd never want to make love again. I couldn't even give myself an orgasm and for the first time in my life I faked when I was with my partner. Then it reached the stage when I actually had an aversion to making love altogether. He's a doctor, luckily, and he kept saying to me, 'Don't worry – this is normal. You'll feel sexy again one day and I don't want to lose you anyway, even if you don't.' He was an absolute darling and although I didn't quite believe him, I hoped it would come back. I did all the right things like eating a healthy diet with lots of vegetables and fruit and exercising each day, which made me feel better generally. I listened to my husband and stopped worrying about my non-existent libido. It took a couple of years and then suddenly I'd have an erotic dream, or catch myself thinking about sex again. I don't get wet any more, but as long as we use lots of lubricant then it's all back to normal. Actually I think my orgasms are even better than they were before – maybe because I value them so much now, they're very special!

Hormone fluctuation can have such a big impact on our moods and sex drive that it's easy to think we're at its mercy. But there's a lot we can do to help our bodies minimise both the hormonal disruption and its effect on our bodies and minds, including our sex drive and capacity for pleasure. My biggest advice from my own experience, is don't give up on sex if hormones submerge your sex drive; keep in touch with your sensuality, even if you're completely off sex, by stroking and massaging yourself or, if possible, having your partner or a masseur give you a massage of some kind.

Massage helped me to become orgasmic: Tracy's story

Reflexology helped keep me feeling sensual, and while having a head massage one day, the thought came into my head that I'd like to go home and masturbate. I did and, with no expectation as I'd never had an orgasm and certainly didn't think I would then, had my first climax.

Whatever your hormones are up to, you are still a sexual, sensual woman. Believe it and you'll encourage your hormones to hurry up and motivate you to enjoy having sex again and to become orgasmic.

Is hormone replacement therapy (HRT) a good idea?

Many women find HRT very helpful in alleviating bothersome menopausal symptoms like overheating and sudden hot flushes, as well as regulating mood swings and tiredness, all of which can make sex seem undesirable. I must point out that certain health risks begin increasing from the earliest days of taking HRT – breast cancer, for instance. However, while many doctors consider short-term use, one to two years, is suitable for alleviating unacceptable menopausal symptoms, longterm use is generally considered inadvisable because of the increased health risk it carries. Moods, tiredness and thermostat (see Adjust your thermostat on page 223) problems will disappear within a year or two of the menopause anyway. If your vagina is persistently dry and the tissues fragile, your doctor may suggest you consider using a vaginally applied oestrogen gel, ring or pessary to help on an occasional basis. If this isn't recommended or you yourself are uncomfortable with the risk, the easiest remedy is to find a lubricant you like (see Useful Resources on page 242) and get into the habit of applying some if ever you feel dry and before and during lovemaking.

An alternative that many claim eases menopausal symptoms is natural progesterone and, although at the time of writing there is little scientific evidence that it works, many women who use it believe it does. Others swear by nutritional supplements, homeopathic or other complementary therapies.

As new research and discoveries are continually being made, I recommend consulting your doctor *and* researching holistic treatments for the latest comprehensive information and advice.

HRT helped me regain my sex drive: Jill's story

Before I went on HRT, menopausal symptoms were putting me right off sex. If we did make love, I'd want my partner to come really quickly – I just wanted to go to sleep and I didn't have an orgasm for months. My partner got fed up with me always refusing him and, on the few times we did make love, not having orgasms like I used to. Eventually he left me, convinced I'd gone off him. I was devastated and didn't think I'd ever meet anyone else. Because I was getting so tired and forgetful, I couldn't even be bothered to self-pleasure. In the end, my doctor prescribed HRT and within days I felt like my old self again. I started going out more, my vivacity came back and to my amazement I found men were still attracted to me. I had three lovers over a period of about four years, and then I met someone very special and we want to stay together forever.

The sex is as good now as it was in my fertile years. It's just that when I was menopausal, pre-HRT, I had no energy or desire to start or persevere through to orgasm. Now I have and I do. I've tried coming off HRT because my doctor advised me to, but all the old symptoms came back. The vaginal forms of HRT are designed to help only with dryness and unsuppleness, which weren't my problem, so there was no point in going on those. I told my doctor I knew the health risks and accepted them as, to me, sexual enjoyment is worth it.

Can HRT increase your sex drive and ability to have orgasms?
While it is possible for HRT, in some forms and circumstances, to increase natural lubrication and encourage the vaginal tissues to retain or regain their elasticity and strength, it doesn't directly increase sex drive or enjoyment of sex. However, if because of taking HRT you stop having hot flushes, your vagina feels more comfortable so you can once again accommodate penetration and you're not tired any more, you're pretty likely to enjoy sex a lot more and thus be orgasmic too.

But our response to hormones depends on whether there are any sensitive hormone receptors on or in the cells, the levels of your own hormone production and the strength of the hormones in the HRT. Then there are medical and dietary considerations and the question of whether the receptors are active or inactive. There is also some evidence that the balance between different hormones may affect their potency as they may work synergistically. In other words, it's mind-bogglingly complicated!

I agree with the medics' advice that it's best not to use oral HRT long term and to bear in mind that even intra-vaginal oestrogen products have some risk. The most important thing is to find a way of keeping your vagina well moisturised, elastic and robust. Even if you're not bothered about having penetrative sex, this is important for your own personal comfort generally, and so that you can have an internal examination without soreness, and also so that you can enjoy sexual pleasure in whichever ways you choose.

Looking after your vagina is part of looking after yourself. Love your body, love yourself, love your sex life and you give yourself the best possible chance of becoming and being orgasmic. See also the section on vaginismus and tightness on page 174 for advice on helping your body avoid or minimise the effects of unsettled hormones.

Keeping your vagina stretchy

Once past the menopause, if we don't have intercourse or use a dildo regularly, the vagina will lose it's stretchiness and we may find it's become difficult or impossible when we do next want to. If this has happened to you and you want to be able to enjoy penetration again, you may be able to gradually regain the suppleness, flexibility and stretchiness of your vagina. Clearly, you're not going to enjoy intercourse if you're sore, which you will be if your vagina – especially the entrance – has become too small for penetration, so don't even think about it until you're confident you're sufficiently stretchy again.

Practise on your own for a while, at first – with plenty of lubricant, of course – just stretching the vaginal entrance by inserting one finger until that's easy, then two, then with the two widening the opening. Once two fingers are really easy, try with a small dildo, not more than two or three centimetres or so at first and then, day by day, go a bit further in, until it once again becomes easy and you're sure you'll be able to have intercourse comfortably. Practise also pelvic floor exercises (see page 119).

Ideally it's a good idea to practise the exercises well before the menopausal years and continue them during and afterwards to completely avoid the possibility of losing vaginal elasticity.

Depression

Loss of desire, diminished arousal and the ability or even the wish to climax are frequent symptoms of depression and, as they can themselves cause or aggravate depression, it can become a self-perpetuating cycle. We need to do something to break the cycle, reach out to happiness, move towards it, pull it to us – and at the same time give physical pleasure and joy a chance to revive. As you do so, another circle comes into being. An enjoyable sex life gives happiness, and feeling good tends to make you feel sexy and sensual.

When we're depressed, sensation is muted. It may feel as though it's gone down just a notch or two or plummeted dramatically.

I didn't want to have sex: Chloe's story

It felt as though someone had turned on the dimmer switch. Everything was grey, as though slightly fogged. I wanted to blow the mist away, put the lights back on. For a while, sex was a welcome relief – it made me feel real again. But then it became more and more of an effort to get aroused until pretty soon I found I couldn't reach orgasm at all. My partner did his best to help me – we tried everything we could think of, but it was no good. In the end, I felt sorry for him and began to fake it. He was a bit suspicious, I think, but rather relieved anyway, I suppose, because it took the onus off him. I thought, is this it? For the rest of my life I'm going to have to fake orgasms, and I'll never get back a feeling of sexual wholeness? It was as though my body and mind had turned against me and perversely taken sexual pleasure away from me. It made me feel more wretched than anything.

Everything loses its edge when you're down. Things don't taste the same, favourite paintings or other beautiful things cease to thrill you, people seem duller – or you feel you're dull around them. And you're probably not as sexy as you used to be. It could be you don't want to make love at all, and/or when you do it lacks conviction or enthusiasm. Even those who are and continue to be orgasmic tend to find the pleasure is diminished and others stop climaxing altogether. And when you lose a fundamental source of pleasure, such a joyous expression of your sexuality and sensuality, it's even more depressing.

At this stage, it's easy to forget the depression came first and to seek solutions for the sexual problem. But with the best will – and counsellor – in the world that's not going to be resolved until the depression and it's underlying causes are.

Take a holistic approach to depression because there are so many possible causes and routes to healing. Even mild depression can have a dramatic effect on desire, arousal and the ability to climax so if you value your sex life as well as your general well-being, it's essential to find out what's making you feel down and what you can do to resolve it.

It could be something as simple as missing out on certain nutrients or daylight, for example, so that your hormone levels aren't balanced. So the first thing you should do is read the section below on your diet to make sure you are giving your body and mind a good foundation for the overall well-being that enables you to take pleasure in your life.

Is what we eat making us happy or miserable?

If you're depressed, although you have a good diet, you may need to look at increasing your consumption of natural foods that are known to specifically enhance our moods:

The amino acid tryptophan is one of the keys to the production of serotonin. It's found in many of our most common protein sources so it is easy to get plenty of – especially lamb, beef, chicken (particularly liver), seafood, pumpkin and sesame seeds and peanuts and Brazil nuts, dairy and soya products. To allow and maximise the effects of tryptophan on serotonin production, the body needs a supply of carbohydrates. This is fascinating because it explains why we sometimes crave chocolate or other comfort foods made of flour and sugar – they don't just make us feel better because they taste good, they actually allow us to feel better by keeping serotonin levels high and well-balanced.

But there's a bit of catch-22 situation to beware of – stuffing ourselves with too much sugar and flour can make us feel heavy as it gives us too many calories and slows down our metabolism, or results in a see-saw of a high just after eating followed by a crash in mood. So the best way to combine the protein foods containing tryptophan with the carbohydrate necessary for its take-up is to choose complex carbohydrates found in wholegrain products, potatoes including their skins, bananas and other fruit which slowly release their sugars.

Phenylalanine, another amino acid, is turned into tyrosine by our bodies, which in turn becomes dopa and then the dopamine that contributes to a feeling of contentment and peace. Again, it's found in many protein foods and especially those mentioned above containing tryptophan. Lima beans, chickpeas, almonds and walnuts are also good sources. And, once again, eating carbohydrates at the same time or within an hour or two facilitates their useful absorption.

A deficiency of folic acid may cause or worsen depression. Rich sources of folic acid are found in green leafy vegetables, pumpkins, carrots and apricots, avocado pears, wholewheat flour, eggs and liver.

A lack of vitamin B6 can inhibit production of mood neurotransmitters, causing or increasing depression. Wheatgerm and bran, cabbage, beef, eggs, offal, black strap molasses and brewer's yeast are all good sources of this.

It's a very basic but rarely mentioned fact that sluggish digestion and constipation can mean you feel bloated, heavy and generally uncomfortable mentally and physically – all of which can make you feel more depressed than ever and anything but sexy. If you are regular on a daily basis, or every other day, that's fine – skip the next few lines. But if several days go by or you have to strain or take laxatives, you could well be feeling less desire, and as congestion in the lower bowel can slow down the arousal curve too, it could be the reason or one of the reasons you're not climaxing.

The remedy is simple – introduce or step up the amount of roughage in your diet. Eat plenty of fresh vegetables, fruit and wholefoods, including the classic natural aids to digestion: figs, spinach, cabbage and linseeds (crush these and introduce them to your diet slowly – a teaspoon a day mixed into muesli, with plenty of liquid, at first, gradually increasing to two dessertspoonfuls will do wonders for your digestion, your skin and your general health).

It's important to note that although you might think an easy way of getting enough of these amino acids and vitamins would be to take ready-made supplements, it's much more effective to consume the relatively smaller amounts naturally by way of the food you eat. And don't consume any food excessively – many foods, however good for us in average portions, are not good for us if overeaten. As in most things – moderation in anything we eat is a sensible guideline.

Is counselling helpful when you're depressed?

I have two friends who sought counselling when they were at a low ebb and they both say their counsellor saved their lives. Mostly, counselling isn't as dramatically successful as this, as not everyone who sees a counsellor is suicidal or anywhere near it. But your counsellor can definitely help you to find the causes of your depression and make you feel better if you are willing to work with them.

To those who have tried counselling and decry it, I'd suggest they weren't ready or willing enough, or simply didn't find the right counsellor – someone they respected, felt safe with, could work with and, importantly, who inspired them to get better. Learning about ourselves and how we can function better in all aspects of our lives takes attention, energy and positivity. You only need tiny amounts of each of these to get going and good counselling will generate future supplies. So just tell yourself, 'Yes, I'm going to book my first appointment with a counsellor who I think I can relate to; yes I'm going to work the way he or she wants; yes, I want it to work.' That's all — a session at a time.

Can I take the self-help route out of depression?

Always seek your doctor's advice in the first instance. But yes, you can help yourself too, and it's important to remember all the different ways we can pull ourselves out of depression or at least keep hold of the thought that we will come out of it in time.

I was always unhappy: Lisa's story

My boyfriend was fed up with me being miserable, hardly ever wanting sex and not climaxing if we did. Eventually he said he couldn't go on with the relationship if I didn't do something about it. I love him and didn't want to lose him, so I decided to have a go at resolving my recurrent depression myself. I read some very good books and knew that a lot of the suggestions and strategies would or might be helpful, but the problem was my depression would swamp my best intentions. That's the trouble with depression – you don't feel like doing anything, even the things that you know would make you feel better.

Lisa's solution was to make several copies of a list of the key strategies she could choose from when she was depressed. She pinned one in her bedroom and one on the door of the fridge:

When I felt down, my gut reaction used to be to go to bed, or to eat. Once I made the decision that I needed to do something about my depression, I'd do something from the list instead, however bad I felt.

It's vital to remember that however bad we feel, we still have the power to change this, reminding ourselves firmly that doing any of the things on the list will rid ourselves of that awful gloom and despondency. The thing is, it will work, whereas sleeping or lying about the place doing nothing or eating when you're not hungry just prolongs the misery. It's important to eat the right things too – eat badly and you'll feel bad; eat well and it boosts morale and helps your body balance hormones better as well as increasing all those feel-good chemicals like serotonin.

Sex drive diminishes with the more depressed you get, then causes relationship problems just to make everything worse. When I was down, the last thing I wanted to do was make love, so my partner was worried that I'd gone off him or he'd done something wrong. Then I'd feel pressured and get annoyed – it's another downward spiral. If you're depressed, you need to do something about it to restore your equilibrium and your sex life. Make that plan – just do it!

Here's a list of strategies that work for many. Add anything that makes you feel better and pick one or more things to do whenever you feel you're on the downward slide:

- Eat something nutritious, delicious and light: It may help to make a list of what you'll eat at every meal because otherwise it may be all too easy to snack on something sugary and fatty that will make you feel worse.

- Exercise: Going for a walk, for instance, works wonders — the exercise releases feel-good hormones and the air and light make you feel good too.
- Dance: Put some upbeat music on and bop your heart out. Dance like nobody's watching — it will give you a huge boost.
- Laugh: Did you know that even pretend laughter makes you feel terrific? Just laugh as if you really were laughing and see what happens. It will feel very strange to be laughing for no reason — but it's infectious! The more you laugh, the more you'll want to laugh and you'll feel much better afterwards. You could, of course, have fun with friends swapping jokes, or watch a comedy.
- Practise thinking positively: The trick is to replace any negative thought with something positive. Positive thinking is just a habit and can be as easily chosen as negativity. It will transform your life and wash depression away.
- Clean something or clear clutter: Pick a chore and do it. Something as simple as sorting a file, mopping the kitchen floor or throwing away a pile of old magazines could uplift your mood. It probably works by re-affirming that you are in charge.
- Do something towards looking good — wash your

hair, put something pretty on, paint your nails, whatever. Taking care of your appearance takes care of your whole well-being.

- Think of someone you love and in your mind give him or her a hug. Better still, if possible, give them a hug for real. Let the love engulf and energise you.
- Do something nice for someone else. Spontaneous acts of kindness feel good.

You may, however, feel so depressed that none of the above helps.

Nothing made me happy: Chloe's story

I couldn't motivate myself to do anything positive – even reading a book about depression seemed like an impossible task. I went to the doctor and cried my way through the appointment after telling him that I didn't even enjoy sex any more and was unable to climax. He recommended counselling but suggested that I was at such a low ebb that it would be sensible to take medication to enable me to take in what the counsellor said and work with her to find out what was behind my depression. He said

that once I was feeling better, the counsellor could
refer me if necessary to a specialist in sex therapy.
As it turned out, it was the counsellor's specialty so
I didn't have to see anyone else.

Chloe found that childhood issues she'd convinced herself were not a problem were sabotaging her present
happiness. Through a mixture of recognition, forgive-
ness and understanding and cognitive therapy, she
overcame her problems and, with help from her doctor,
gradually came off the medication.

Although I felt so much better, I still had virtually no
libido but my counsellor said that this could be a
symptom of the medication I was taking. It seems she
was right because once I was off it, I felt sexier than I
had for ages – or ever, if I'm honest. It took a while to
climax again, but I no longer faked and found I really
enjoyed sex anyway. My partner, now that he understood me better and I guess because he was proud of
me for having the courage to heal, became very tender and gentle. Suddenly sex was sensuous and
whatever he did seemed to me to be more erotic
than ever before. When I had my first orgasm, I was
stunned and he was even more pleased than me!

It's a good idea for everyone not to take good sex for granted, especially when you're depressed. As mentioned elsewhere in this book, it's easy to find you don't bother to make love regularly even though you love it when you do.

Is medication really necessary?

Not always, but often it's very helpful and sometimes it's essential. Without it, as Chloe's doctor pointed out, someone who is severely depressed may not be able to focus on the counsellor's thoughts, let alone her own, during sessions. If you can deal constructively with your depression without it, that's good, but if not, think of it as one of the positive strategies in your holistic list.

There are several natural remedies available from the pharmacist or health shop that may help. Complementary therapies can also be useful, even if it's a placebo effect. For instance, although there is no scientific proof that homeopathy has a physical effect, many find it works for them. Psychosomatic or not, in my view if it succeeds in prising open the clutches of depression and has no side effects, it's irrelevant why or how it works. Unless you find your depression responds to and clears with self-help strategies, see your doctor – he or she has the expertise to assess whether counselling, medication or a combination of the two is most apt and can refer you to a counsellor and prescribe medication as necessary.

Most of us need to feel good in ourselves and about ourselves (and about our partner if we're in a relationship) to feel positively sexy and to have orgasms easily. With the right help, we can cure depression and stop ourselves from being besieged by it again.

The pill and other contraceptives

The contraceptive pills – oestrogen only and oestrogen/progestogen combined – can certainly have an effect on sex drive and the ability to get aroused and have orgasms. The effect can be slight or dramatic and can vary dramatically from woman to woman. Of those who do experience a change, most find their libido and capacity for pleasure decreases, but many find the exact opposite and feel sexier all round.

So if you're not on the pill, are in your fertile years and have never had orgasms or have stopped having them, taking the pill might have no effect on your desire for sex, arousability and orgasmability, or it could increase or decrease them. But as the chances of an increase aren't great, no one would advise you to give the pill a try with the sole purpose that it might help. However, if you are going on the pill anyway for contraceptive protection or, as it's sometimes prescribed, to balance an erratic menstrual cycle, you may find your sex drive and pleasure increase – either as an effect of the hormones in the pill or because, safe from the possibility of conceiving or freed from menstrual cycle problems, you're more relaxed about having sex.

Try changing your contraception: Stella's story

I went on the pill at college. Although I always insisted on condoms when I had sex for protection against STIs, I didn't trust them as a contraceptive and wanted to feel secure I wouldn't get pregnant. I still fancied men and fell in love like I did before I was on the pill, but the pleasure factor when we had sex lost its edge. It just wasn't as good. Although I didn't climax the few times I'd made love pre-pill, I got very close and was sure I soon would – you know that 'I'm coming' feeling? Although it still felt nice on the pill, I didn't get to that on the brink thing at all. I told my doctor and he suggested changing to another still reliable contraceptive that wouldn't affect my hormones and sex drive. He recommended a diaphragm and though my friends think it's old-fashioned I really like it. All the feelings I'd originally had came back and it wasn't long before I learnt how to take myself over 'the brink' and have orgasms. I still insisted on using condoms while I was having casual sex, but now I've settled down with my boyfriend, we don't need to worry about STIs any more.

Good side effects from the pill: Lisa's story

I've taken the pill for years with only good side effects. My GP checks my blood pressure and heart rate regularly and they're always normal so she's happy to keep prescribing it. The benefits are my skin's clear whereas before I was always getting spots, especially the week before my periods, and I don't get cramps any more. Sex? It's no better, no worse – I enjoy it just like I always have. It's made no difference to orgasms either – sometimes I have them, sometimes I don't.

So it depends on how the pill suits you. If you think you might be more orgasmic if you went on or came off the pill, talk it over with your doctor.

If you're on the progestogen-only pill, most of the above applies, but a different possible side effect is that some women experience bleeding or spotting between periods. If this is happening to you, it might easily be affecting your sexual feelings and you should tell your doctor and discuss alternatives.

Contraceptive injections and patches make sexual side effects less likely than either kind of oral pill.

Other contraceptives

Diaphragm, Dutch cap, various types of coil, condoms, the rhythm and withdrawal methods – it's very much a personal choice. If you find a method you're happy with, then the method itself is unlikely to affect your sex drive or pleasure. If your chosen method worries you because it's uncomfortable for you or even for your partner, or you fear it's unreliable, it can, as the following personal experience shows, have a big effect on your orgasmability.

Contraception is an individual thing: Stephanie's story

After I mistakenly got pregnant and then miscarried, I realised I needed a reliable method of contraception than the hit-and-miss one we'd been using, which was easy to forget. I didn't want to take the pill so my doctor suggested and fitted me with a coil. It didn't suit me at all – I had horrendously heavy periods and often experienced sharp, shooting pains throughout the month. My husband didn't like it either as he said he could feel it and it was scratchy. All in all, it felt like an alien intrusion in my body and I didn't have a single orgasm while it was there. I was really disappointed as a couple of friends are fine with theirs, and though I persevered in the hope things would improve, they didn't. It put us both off intercourse completely and we soon stopped making loving at all. I guess that meant it was a very effective contraceptive indeed! My doctor removed it and suggested I give chemical contraception a go, but a patch rather than the pill. It has no side effects for me and we're now having some great sex. Whether it's the relief that all is well now or whatever, I'm more orgasmic than I've ever been. It doesn't happen every time – but much more often than it used to. I'd advise everyone to persevere in finding a method they personally like – it's such an individual thing.

If you're not happy with your contraception or you're worried about the lack of it, it could reduce your sexual desire, arousal and enjoyment and orgasms are likely to be the first casualty. So being comfortable and feeling safe with your method is crucial to your orgasmability and it's certainly worth persevering until you find the one that's right for you. Question friends, your doctor, the Family Planning Clinic and books on the subject so you have all the facts at your fingertips and some personal opinions to help you choose. Don't be afraid to change the method – it's your body, you have a perfect right to look after its well-being. Doctor's sometimes advise trying a particular brand of chemical contraceptive for at least three months, but if you are in discomfort or pain, go back and ask if you can stop taking it immediately. If this is unwise, do so at the end of the current cycle. Contraception shouldn't hurt and if it does, it's not right for you so find another method that doesn't.

Fertility – questions and difficulties

For many women, the enjoyment of sex and orgasms is tied up with fertility, and problems with it are a much more common cause of anorgasmia than is usually noted. My heart goes out to you if you longed for children but are unable to have them. I understand how difficult or impossible it may seem that you will be able to accept the situation and focus on all the current and potential good in your life. Most women consider having children at some stage, and although more are deciding not to, of those that do want to go ahead, many feel it's a major purpose of their life. To then find you can't have a baby can be devastating. Many emotions are involved, including, for many, a multifaceted sense of loss – loss of their vision of how their life would be and of their anticipated role as mother and one day grandmother, and thus a deep sense of losing their identity too. But I urge you to hold on to the fact that your life can be good in a different way and equally fulfilling and enjoyable in its own right. You'll find suggested books to help in the Useful Resources section on page 242. But this is a book about orgasms – so let's get back to sex...

As the emotions consciously or subconsciously connected with infertility are so complex and powerful, they may drastically affect your attitude to sex.

I felt sad and childless: Sally's story

Sex seemed pointless once we'd gone through all the tests and treatments and been told we would almost certainly never have children. My husband was sympathetic for a while, but soon expected me to accept it and move on. I just couldn't. One day I almost bit his head off when he tried to seduce me and I realised I needed to get help. The counsellor believed in a cognitive approach, which meant working out and using practical ways to move on and enjoy life and sex again. But she also helped me to look at why I so desperately wanted my own babies and I learnt it wasn't only a physical drive, it was all about my childhood. My mother's view was that a woman's only worthwhile if she's a good mother. She also thought the only reason for sex was to produce babies. Finding out that I wasn't mad and there were very real psychological and physical reasons for my feelings and antipathy towards sex was like the lights going on again. It took a lot of practice, but I've learnt to rationalise the truth: I don't have to have kids to be a valuable person or to be happy and lovable; sex is a wonderful thing in its own right. I also began to think positively about the possibilities for enjoying life and now I'm living them. I learnt, too, to see sex in a new light – as an expression of our love for each other and as a pure, unadulterated source of physical and emotional pleasure and joy.

Sally changed her attitude from thinking of herself as a sad, childless woman to a happy woman who loves life and who happens not to have children, and everyone can do this if they want to and are willing to do what it takes like Sally so courageously did. Counselling isn't easy when complex and deep-rooted emotions are involved, but it can be empowering and cathartic. If you decide to go this route, I recommend seeing a psychosexual counsellor, as their general experience should be comprehensive in addition to their specialisation in sexual issues.

If you had orgasm difficulties before the fears about infertility started, then learning techniques to give you the greatest sexual pleasure and potential for orgasms will be extremely helpful. (See chapter 3 and chapter 5.)

The idea of finding or designing your own fantasy as described below in the section on the effect of contraceptive-induced infertility could work for you too, revolutionising your enjoyment of sex and orgasms which in turn will give your self-esteem and enjoyment of life generally a powerful boost.

Even using highly effective contraceptives, for instance the pill or a cap, coil or diaphragm, can have a big psychological impact on your desire and orgasmability levels.

I can't come any more: Belinda's story

For me, fertility was sexy. Lovemaking with my part-ner was exciting because of the possibility of creating a new life. When he was about to come, I'd have a surge of arousal and climax when he came or within seconds afterwards. It's a bit of a paradox because although I loved that feeling of 'maybe this time I'll conceive,' we don't actually want children. We wouldn't be good parents and anyway, we like our life together just as it is. Someone said we were selfish – but surely it's no more selfish to not have kids because you don't want them than to have them because you do? So I have no issues about not feeling like a real woman unless I'm a mother, or anything like that – it's purely and simply that I miss the excitement when Graham's about to ejaculate. It isn't the same any more and though I still love sex, I can't make myself come. He gets fed up with hold-ing his climax back while I try to, and in the end, every time, I realise there's no hope so I pretend I've got there.

I asked Belinda if there was a psychological reason other than the excitement factor and after pondering this for a while, she said that she did like the idea of being fertile as it had made her feel very feminine and fecund. She said she couldn't help a slight concern, though, that perhaps she wasn't, as they'd made love for several months without conceiving.

She said that, yes, that as well losing the excitement, she also felt she'd lost the chance to prove that she is really as fertile as she felt. As she and her partner were already accomplished lovers and she had been very orgasmic with him before they started using contraceptives, I suggested developing a fantasy where she was a highly fertile woman in an exotic setting, either chosen by a man specifically to mother his child, or herself choosing and being served by a man specifically as her stud.

At our next session Belinda told me gleefully that she'd had great fun reading some books on women's fantasies for ideas and testing them out while self-pleasuring. She chose the one that turned her on the most and, after personalising it, found she'd climax for real when her character in the fantasy did. She then practised using it while making love with her partner and was thrilled it worked.

Chapter 8

Why am I Still Not Orgasming?

Adjust your thermostat…

It sounds like a small consideration, but it could have a big impact on whether or not you have an orgasm. If you're freezing cold, you'll be unhappy and less likely to feel sexy. And if you're way too hot, the last thing you want to do is have sex and get even more uncomfortable.

Too hot to handle: Lucy's story

I've always had a tendency to be too hot and rarely feel the cold but my partner's the opposite. Within a few seconds of cuddling I'd be boiling and push him away. He couldn't understand because, of course, he loves getting close up and warmer, so he'd be hurt. It was only when this came out in passing as we talked to you, and you pointed out to us that I was unlikely to come when, (a) I didn't want to make love in the first place because I was too hot, and, (b) I never got fully aroused – again because I was too hot. We solved the problem by keeping the house several degrees cooler. He puts a sweater on when he's at home and he loves making love because he gets nice and warm despite the cool bedroom, which means I don't overheat! He's also realised it's best not to wrap himself round me when we're getting aroused and by keeping some distance between us until we have intercourse I can enjoy getting really aroused and at long last I'm having orgasms. It wasn't just the temperature factor – we both learnt to improve our technique, but it definitely made our love life much more viable.

Even women who are cold mortals when young can find themselves besieged by hot flushes during the menopause.

The menopause made me too hot: Ella's story

Suddenly I'd feel as though I was blazing. I'd go bright pink and would sweat profusely. My metabolism altered, no doubt about it, and whereas before I'd loved snuggling up to my husband in bed, now I couldn't bear him too near me. I totally lost desire and the ability to climax. Then I changed my diet, began to exercise every day at the gym and swam too. I gave up my beloved wine and apart from a couple of half-shot lattes in the morning, stopped drinking coffee too. Almost immediately I started to feel more like my old self and stopped fending my husband off.

A self-help campaign like this can let you sail through the menopause. Your sex drive might still not be the same as before for a year or two, but just bear in mind it will come back once your body adjusts if you encourage and pay attention to it, and so your orgasmability.

If, on the other hand, you're the kind of person who goes blue with cold when the temperature dips, you need to exercise more. Once you get your circulation going, you soon get warm and feel vibrantly sensual. When you're cold, your body goes into hibernation mode, stilling senses and slowing sexual responses.

As in most aspects of life, balance is the key to happiness and sensuality. Know yourself, notice changes in your metabolism and work out a plan to adjust or manage the new tendency to be hot or cold. If it's out of control, it could be sabotaging your orgasmability so check it out.

Medication

If you are taking any kind of medication, check with your doctor whether it could be affecting your sex drive. If it's possible that it is, and your condition still needs to be treated, he or she will consider whether it's possible to change your prescription. Loss of interest in sex can, for instance, be a side effect of some of the medication used for treating depression, and of beta blockers for high blood pressure.

The importance of sleep

Maybe sleeping well doesn't spring to mind as being one of the essentials for being orgasmic, but for most of us, it is. When we're tired, our minds and bodies ache to shut down and probably do in some measure even when sleep is impractical. Our sex drive needs energy, alertness, willingness and enthusiasm for the physical component to kick-start and gain speed, but these are the very things that drain from us when we're weary.

Managing fatigue so it doesn't scupper your sex life

When you're so tired all you want to do is sleep, it's probably because you need to. If you're so exhausted you don't want to make love, don't – you'll only resent your partner if it's his idea, and if you're on your own and decide to give yourself pleasure, you'll simply fall asleep. To climax you can be energised or deeply relaxed but this doesn't mean sleepy. You need to be fully aware of the sensations and if the longing to sleep is pulling you into oblivion, even with the best intention and technique in the world, you're unlikely to climax.

So get some sleep. If it's bedtime, set the alarm clock half an hour earlier so you can have sex when you wake up. Just before you go to sleep tell yourself, 'I will sleep soundly and wake feeling refreshed, full of life again and keen to make love and have an orgasm.' Your subconscious will store the suggestion for it to happen for real on waking. You may need to help your conscious mind if you immediately revert to a resistance to this and decide you are still too sleepy by remembering your decision to make love in the morning and thinking, 'Come on, let's just do it!'

If you feel too exhausted earlier in the evening or during the day to make love, by all means have a catnap. Sleep for a maximum of 30 minutes but no more because if you sleep for too long, you won't sleep well that night and it will set up a cycle of a poor night's sleep and ongoing fatigue.

Though this will keep your sex life going through times when fatigue's unavoidable – like when you've a young baby who's not yet sleeping through the night, for instance – generally by far the best way to be full of energy, wide awake and sexy when you want is to have a good seven or eight hours' sleep at a stretch. It's all about recharging. When you're asleep, your body and mind are busy digesting food and facts, healing and renewing cells and tissues. In the process your sex drive is revitalised, so much so that it's common to have an erotic dream just before you wake up. If this happens to you, 'hold' the feelings and the sensations and keeping them in mind, make love for real.

Becoming a good sleeper...

Again, if establishing a regular sleep pattern is something you only dream of, there are books on the subject to help (see Useful Resources on page 242).

Go to bed seven hours (the average good night's sleep) before you intend to get up, so if you set the alarm for seven, get into bed at midnight. Try to get off to sleep by doing something peaceful like meditating or reading. Don't fret if you don't sleep. Just lie there, relax and enjoy the rest. Do not get up – just stay put and wait it out. At seven when your alarm goes off, get up, even if you haven't slept very well.

If you didn't sleep much or even at all, don't be tempted to sleep during the day – not even a catnap. Within a night or two, your mind will suss it has to use those seven hours to sleep and will do so. After a week assess the situation. If you're still a bit wakeful during the seven hours in bed, then reduce them to six or six and a half. If you sleep right through to be woken by the alarm, extend the time to seven and a half or eight hours. We all vary a bit but most of us need somewhere between six and eight hours. Our personal need can change at different life stages, too. I used to need eight but nowadays only need six and a half or seven, depending how busy I am. So be flexible and adjust your time in bed as needed.

Other ways to wind down before bed are to watch something undemanding on the TV, for instance, or drink a warm, milky drink or a chamomile tea – this will make you feel tranquil and prime your mind and body to start relaxing and prepare for a good night's sleep.

Insomnia ruined my relationship: Nicky's story

I used to suffer from insomnia and I'd get myself hyped up for work and then crash when I got home. My partner would try to make love and sometimes I'd feel so tired I'd literally push him away – I had no energy for it and no desire whatsoever. It wasn't that I didn't find him attractive. True, I'd never had an orgasm and always faked it but when we did make love, it was pleasant enough – I just lived on tiredness and went off it completely. He ditched me, understandably enough, and when, after a couple of months of initial excitement with a new boyfriend I found I was becoming just as tired and reluctant to have sex as before, I knew I had to do something about it. I cut the time in bed like you advised and got used to sleeping for six hours at first. I immediately began to feel better and have more energy. I still get sleepy after supper, but after a short catnap I'm wide awake and that's when we usually make love, before bedtime so I don't get panicky and think I won't have enough sleep. He thinks I'm funny having a sleep routine but he's glad because we have wonderful sex now two or three times a week and I love it. I've also become orgasmic – mostly because we practise CAT (see page 114) – but I think the fact I'm sleeping so well may also have something to do with it.

I'm sure it did – orgasm takes a lot of energy, both mental and physical– so tiredness tends to shut down our capacity for it. That's partly why we make love such a lot and with so much pleasure on holiday – when we play hard and relax well we sleep like a log and our libido flourishes. But you don't have to be on holiday to sleep well – it's just about getting into a routine. So do it – it will let your sex drive and orgasmability thrive.

Alcohol and drugs

I enjoy a glass of good wine as much as anyone but I know that's my personal limit. Any more and after the initial high which lasts about an hour, I'm sleepy or argumentative, neither of which do much for my sex drive.

Some people can't drink at all without an adverse effect; few can drink more than a glass or two of wine without lowering their sensory reactions and for many a sensitive woman that translates as decreasing their sexuality.

You will have a good idea if alcohol, coffee or another social drug could be affecting your well-being adversely. If this is so, or even possibly so, do reduce or cut out your intake as apt for you as it could also be the reason you're not having orgasms. If addicted to alcohol or drugs, get help coming off them (see Useful Resources on page 242).

Everyone has their own unique metabolism and so we each have our own individual tolerance level. Get to know yours and stick within it.

Freedom from the effect of abuse

When we're abused, the emotional agony isn't just of the moment — it can affect our whole attitude to ourselves, others, life generally and, especially with sexual abuse of course, our sexuality and sex. This personal experience shows how insidious the legacy can be, but how freedom from it can be found.

Dealing with the leftovers of abuse: Hannah's story

I'd never had an orgasm and I didn't know why. My friends said it was easy and began to tease me because I didn't know what they were talking about. They said that when I met the right man, everything would fall into place and it would just happen. But however fanciable my boyfriends were and however aroused I got, it didn't. At first, when many of my partners realised I hadn't come, they'd think it was a challenge and try to get me there. In the end I felt like such a freak that I pretended to boyfriends that I'd started having orgasms and that everything was fine. It wasn't and eventually I went to the sexual health clinic at the general hospital and started seeing a psychosexual therapist.

I found myself telling my therapist about the abuse I'd had from my stepfather when I was a kid. I thought I'd put it all behind me in my determination not to let him affect my life. But all the emotions came welling up – fear, anger and shame – but most of all the shame. She helped me see that I couldn't just pretend it hadn't affected my attitude to sex and helped me work through the issues. I realise I might have to do so throughout my life whenever they came up again but I'm not scared of them any more. The extraordinary thing was that I began to feel compassionate towards myself, and towards boyfriends. I wasn't my stepfather's 'accomplice' and they weren't my stepfather. The counsellor suggested I'd had deepdown resistance to allowing myself to have an orgasm and to letting anyone else give me one. I had my first orgasm on my own, and then masturbated every day for weeks because I was so thrilled. Soon afterwards, I began to have them when I was having sex with my boyfriend. I feel free of the abuse and my stepfather and will never again let the negative emotions about them affect the joy of being orgasmic.

Fear, anger, shame – as Hannah found out, the most difficult thing to deal with is shame. It could be from any abuse – sexual, physical or verbal. Though aware that the abuse was not your fault you may still have a feeling of shame that shadows you. Every woman and every situation is different and this book isn't the place to advise on dealing with negative emotions ensuing from abuse.

If you have suffered abuse and would like to explore its effect on your sex drive and ability to orgasm, I recommend having counselling with a psychologist or psychotherapist qualified and experienced in dealing with sexual problems. They will help you understand the issues and in a sense learn to neutralise negative memories and emotions so that they no longer damage you in the present. You can free your mind, and in so doing, your body. (See the Useful Resources section on page 242 for more information.)

Let go of learnt inhibitions

It doesn't take many times of a mother saying to her small daughter, 'Don't touch yourself there,' for the child to get the idea that masturbation is somehow not right and that sex isn't either. Worse inhibitions are born if you accept the idea from your mother that sex and your genitals are dirty. TV programmes such as *Sex and the City* and documentaries where women frankly and openly discuss sex in explicit detail have helped to tear down taboos and resultant inhibitions still prevalent at the end of the last millennium. But even today women still don't feel equal to men in this area.

If you feel you're inhibited about your body or some aspect of sex, freeing yourself of it could make all the difference to your ability to let yourself go and have orgasms. How should you go about freeing yourself? Once again, talking to a psychosexual counsellor will be helpful. Please don't think a general counsellor will do – without training and practice, few people can comfortably discuss sex in detail with a comparative stranger whereas psychosexual therapists are steeped in the language of sexuality and, totally relaxed, will be good at putting you at your ease and helping you become fluent in talking about sex too. The more you talk, the quicker your inhibitions will dissolve; you'll be able to get to the root of uncomfortable feelings about sex and set about building a healthier attitude and mindset.

I've thrown off my mother's warnings: Daisy's story

Although she had me when she was 18, and is now only 38, my mother has an almost Victorian view of sex. She gets embarrassed if there are sex scenes on TV and once she barged into my room when I was playing with myself and told me I was disgusting and that I mustn't do it again. She's also a misandrist – she was always saying sexist things about men when I was growing up and disliked most of them intensely, especially my father, who, not surprisingly left her. I came to the conclusion that men are just like women – not all good and not all bad but a mixture. But maybe I did take on her feeling that men were sexually gross as I realised early in my teens that I'm not attracted to men and finally accepted I'm gay. But with my first girlfriend, I couldn't throw off the feeling that we were doing something wrong when we made love. I'd get so tense that there was no way I could have an orgasm, even though I'd secretly continued to masturbate since my mother's condemnation of it and could bring myself to climax on my own.

Years later I met an amazing woman and fell in love. I really wanted to give myself completely to the pleasure of lovemaking and orgasm, so I found a qualified sex therapist. We saw her six times and she helped me confront all my inhibitions and lose the idea that having sex and enjoying it was wrong. My partner was wonderful – we didn't have sex for a couple of weeks while we did lots of the body massage 'homework' the counsellor set us. This taught me how to relax, and when we started having sex again, I'd loosened up so much I could at last thoroughly enjoy it. I've become really passionate now, and the sex we have is out of this world. We always climax, sometimes together, sometimes taking turns.

Once again, losing inhibitions is a question of freeing your mind from erroneous beliefs and understanding the truth: sex on your own or with a partner you choose to have it with is normal, natural and good.

A Final Note

I've often found that disinterest in sex and other sexual difficulties follow on from the person's feeling that life's meaningless or that they haven't 'found' themselves, or are missing out on their potential.

It's quite common to lose libido and orgasmability during midlife crisis – and this dissatisfaction with who we are and where we are in our life's path can occur at any time. It's a time when you find yourself questioning, Who am I? What purpose does my life have? Is this how it's always going to be until the end? It is usually assumed that this happens when we're 40- or 50ish, panicking to suddenly realise we're literally halfway through our expected lifespan and may not have many more active years. But in fact similar questions can gather or regroup at any time of our adult lives. If you're in your 20s or 30s, for instance, you may have hit a phase of wondering what you want – *really want* – to do with the rest of your life, realising that what you're doing now is not it. Or if you're heading for or in the third age — 60-plus — you may be thinking of opportunities missed and whether they or new ones can still be grasped to lead to deeper fulfilment and happiness.

This time of questioning often causes anxiety, panic and/or depression as the prospect of change can be frightening. Not only is this likely to depress your sex drive and ability to have orgasms, whatever your age, but if you have a partner, your anxiety may be affecting them and, if so, could be causing relationship difficulties, only adding to the decline in your sex drive.

If this is striking a chord with you, then please start your quest to discover the real you now. I'm talking about the person you sense you are deep down, not a role you might play. Meditation can be very helpful in times of uncertainty and change of direction; talking to a counsellor can also be helpful and inspirational.

Living orgasmically

The path to becoming orgasmic is an eclectic, very individual mixture of physical technique and responses and a positive attitude to sensual and sexual pleasure and fulfilment. Being orgasmic on an ongoing basis is more of the same. Mostly, once you've got the knack on both fronts, it will be automatic. But like all abilities, skills and habits, your sex drive and orgasmability

A Final Note

will need regular maintenance and input. So think of sex often, keep in touch with all your senses, think and live positively.

Most of all, keep a loving attitude to yourself and your sexuality throughout your life. You have the great gift of sensuality. Enjoy it to the full.

Useful Resources

Books

Sex

How Was It For You? Making Sex Much, Much Better by Anne Hooper (Carroll & Brown, 2005)

This informative book is well-written and offers some great advice on how to improve your sex life.

Massage Secrets for Lovers by Andrew Stanway (Carroll & Graf, 2003)

Gives all the tips on how to spice up your sex life with the art of sensual massage.

The Multi-Orgasmic Woman by Mantak Chia and Dr Rachel Carlton Abrams (Rodale, 2005)

Contains great tips for honing your orgasmic skills.

Think Sex by Jenny Hare (Vega, 2001)

I wrote this book because many people forget that good sex starts in the mind.

Women's Pleasure by Rachel Swift (Pan, 1994)

Brilliant for suggesting ways for women to find out what they like in bed.

Fantasy

The Joy of Sexual Fantasy by Andrew Stanway (Carroll & Graf, 1998)

A good starting point if you've not had much experience with fantasy in the past.

Self-esteem

Gael Lindenfield's Self-Esteem Bible: Build Your Confidence Day by Day by Gael Lindenfield (Element, 2004)

Living in the Light by Shakti Gawain (Bantam Doubleday Dell, 1998)

This book changed my life when I first read an earlier edition over a decade ago. It's just the loveliest book — another one I like to re-read.

Remarkable Changes by Jane Seymour (Regan Books, 2003)

Jane Seymour's gentle strength, courage and joie de vivre inspire you to accept change and seek out the new possibilities and opportunities.

You Can Heal Your Life by Louise Hay (Full Circle, 2003)

A treasure for healing and growing your self-esteem. I re-read it every year to remind myself of the wisdom.

Relationships

Creating Love by John Bradshaw (Piatkus,1992)

John Bradshaw's insight into our fears and difficulties with love inspires tremendous understanding, deep healing and greater ability to love and accept love.

Dare to Connect: How to Create Confidence, Trust and Loving Relationships by Susan Jeffers (Piatkus, 2005)

Love by Leo Buscaglia (Souvenir Press, 1984)

Leo Buscaglia was just the most amazing man – he wrote about love so enthusiastically and wisely you wonder how we can ever forget to live lovingly.

Think Love by Jenny Hare (Vega, 2003)

How to let love light up your life.

General

Breaking Free: Help for Survivors of Child Sexual Abuse by Carolyn Ainscough and Kay Toon (Sheldon, 2000)

Freedom from Addiction: The Secret Behind Successful Addiction Busting by Joe Griffin and Ivan Tyrrell (HG Publishing, 2005)

Manage Your Pain by Michael Nicholas, Allan Malloy, Lois Tonkin and Lee Betson (Souvenir Press, 2006)

Overcoming Insomnia and Sleep Problems by Colin A. Espie (Constable and Robinson, 2006)

Vibrators and sex toys

www.annsummers.com
tel: 0845 456 2399

www.bedroompleasures.co.uk
tel: 0800 0751 633

www.sh-womenstore.com
tel: 020 7613 5458

Sex therapy and counselling

British Association for Sexual and Relationship Therapy
www.BASRT.org.uk
tel: 020 8543 2707

Relate, the relationship people
www.relate.org.uk
Log on to the website or see your phone book to find
your local branch.

General counselling

British Association for Counselling and Psychotherapy
www.bacp.co.uk
tel: 0870 443 5252

UK Therapists
www.uktherapists.com

About the Author

Jenny Hare is a psychosexual therapist and counsellor. She has also been *Woman's Weekly's* agony aunt for many years.